CAMBRIDGE LIBRARY COLLECTION

Books of enduring scholarly value

Women's Writing

The later twentieth century saw a huge wave of academic interest in women's writing, which led to the rediscovery of neglected works from a wide range of genres, periods and languages. Many books that were immensely popular and influential in their own day are now studied again, both for their own sake and for what they reveal about the social, political and cultural conditions of their time. A pioneering resource in this area is Orlando: Women's Writing in the British Isles from the Beginnings to the Present (http://orlando.cambridge.org), which provides entries on authors' lives and writing careers, contextual material, timelines, sets of internal links, and bibliographies. Its editors have made a major contribution to the selection of the works reissued in this series within the Cambridge Library Collection, which focuses on non-fiction publications by women on a wide range of subjects from astronomy to biography, music to political economy, and education to prison reform.

England and Her Soldiers

In the preface to this 1859 book Harriet Martineau (1802–76) tells the reader that this 'is not a work of invention' or a 'fancy-piece' and thereby sets the tone for a study that is partly historical and partly sociological. In the writing of the book, Martineau collaborated with another prominent nineteenth-century figure, Florence Nightingale. They wished to gain political support for improvements in military hygiene and health care. Martineau draws on Nightingale's experiences when nursing wounded soldiers during the Crimean War and builds it into a strong narrative that describes the conditions that soldiers experienced in the barracks, in hospitals and on the field. Martineau also focuses on the administration of hygiene and health care in general, and makes practical recommendations as how to improve these areas, by legislation if necessary, so as to ensure the future good health of Britain's armed forces. For more information on this author, see http://orlando.cambridge.org/public/svPeople?person_id=martha

Cambridge University Press has long been a pioneer in the reissuing of out-of-print titles from its own backlist, producing digital reprints of books that are still sought after by scholars and students but could not be reprinted economically using traditional technology. The Cambridge Library Collection extends this activity to a wider range of books which are still of importance to researchers and professionals, either for the source material they contain, or as landmarks in the history of their academic discipline.

Drawing from the world-renowned collections in the Cambridge University Library, and guided by the advice of experts in each subject area, Cambridge University Press is using state-of-the-art scanning machines in its own Printing House to capture the content of each book selected for inclusion. The files are processed to give a consistently clear, crisp image, and the books finished to the high quality standard for which the Press is recognised around the world. The latest print-on-demand technology ensures that the books will remain available indefinitely, and that orders for single or multiple copies can quickly be supplied.

The Cambridge Library Collection will bring back to life books of enduring scholarly value (including out-of-copyright works originally issued by other publishers) across a wide range of disciplines in the humanities and social sciences and in science and technology.

England and Her Soldiers

Harriet Martineau

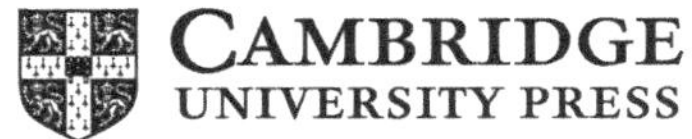

CAMBRIDGE UNIVERSITY PRESS

Cambridge, New York, Melbourne, Madrid, Cape Town, Singapore,
São Paolo, Delhi, Dubai, Tokyo, Mexico City

Published in the United States of America by Cambridge University Press, New York

www.cambridge.org
Information on this title: www.cambridge.org/9781108020565

This edition first published 1859
This digitally printed version 2010

ISBN 978-1-108-02056-5 Paperback

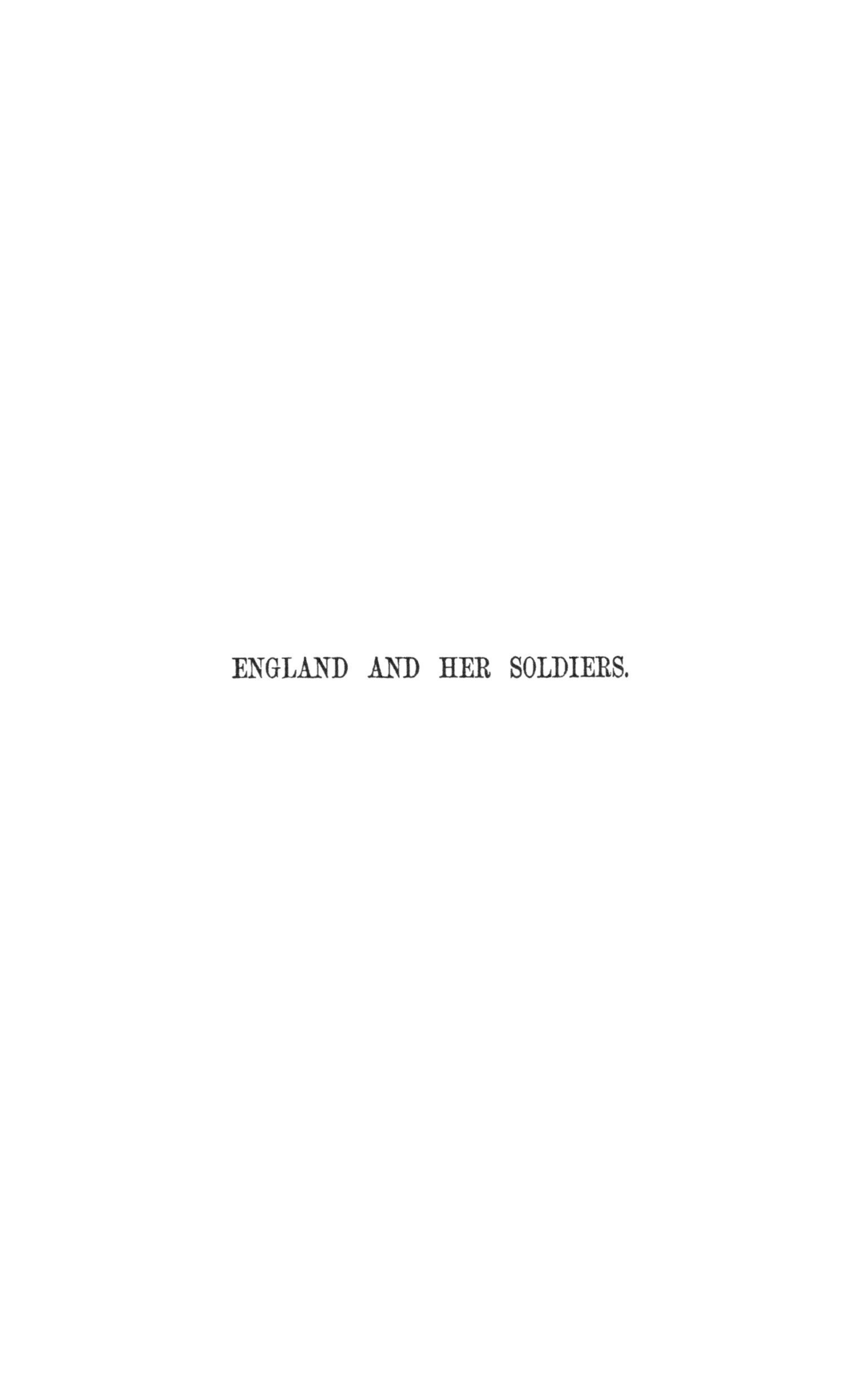

ENGLAND AND HER SOLDIERS.

LONDON
PRINTED BY SPOTTISWOODE AND CO.
NEW-STREET SQUARE

DIAGRAM OF THE CA

IN THE ARMY

2.

APRIL 1855 TO MARCH 1856.

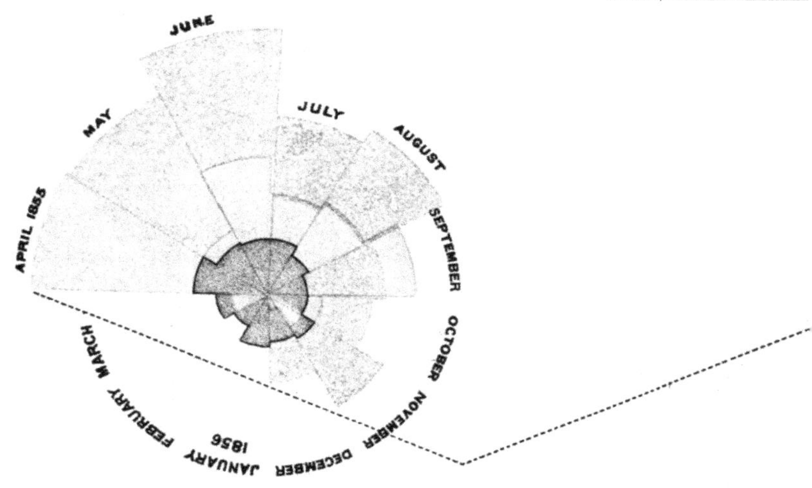

The Areas of the blue, red, & black wedges are each measured from the centre as the common vertex.

The blue wedges measured from the centre of the circle represent area for area the deaths from Preventible or Mitigable Zymotic diseases; the red wedges measured from the centre the deaths from wounds; & the black wedges measured from the centre the deaths from all other causes.

The black line across the red triangle in Nov.r 1854 marks the boundary of the deaths from all other causes during the month.

In October 1854, & April 1855, the black area coincides with the red; in January & February 1855, the blue coincides with the black.

The entire areas may be compared by following the blue, the red & the black lines enclosing them.

SES OF MORTALITY

THE EAST.

1.

APRIL 1854 TO MARCH 1855.

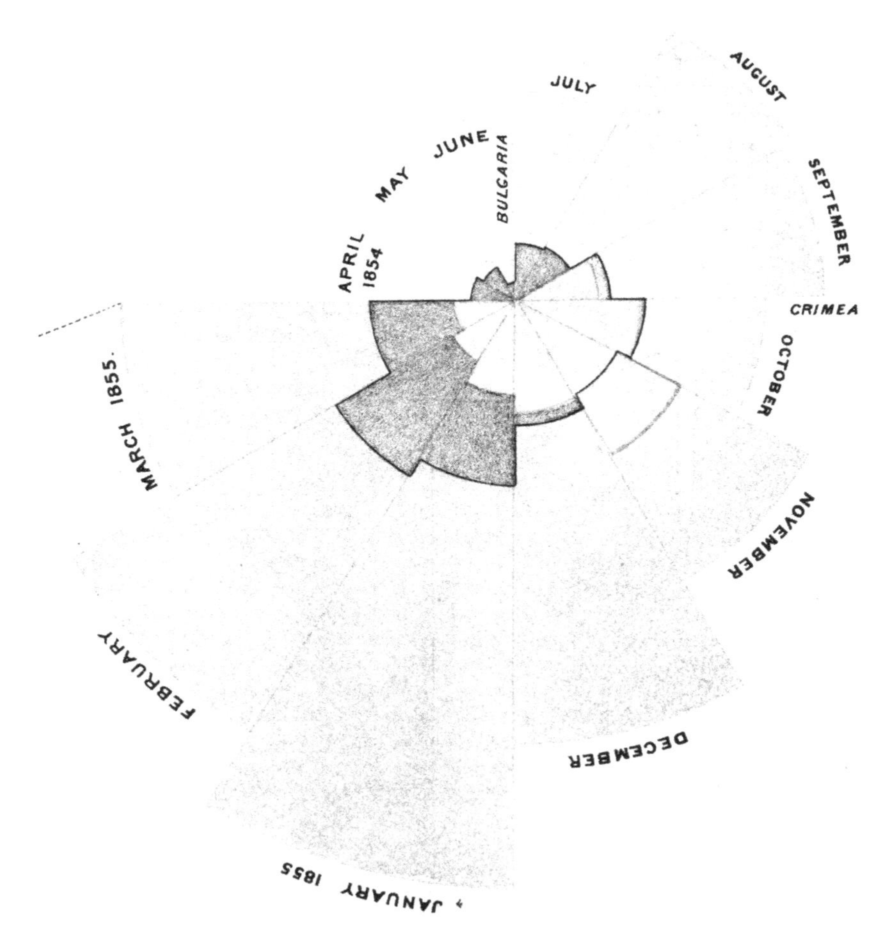

ENGLAND AND HER SOLDIERS.

BY HARRIET MARTINEAU.

"Let me speak proudly.—Tell the Constable
We are but warriors for the working day:
Our gayness, and our gilt, are all besmirched
With rainy marching in the painful field.
There's not a piece of feather in our host
(Good argument, I hope, we shall not fly),
And time hath worn us into slovenry:
But, by the mass, our hearts are in the trim."
KING HENRY V., Act iv. *Scene* 3.

"I know already by your forwardness, that you have deserved rewards and crowns; and we do assure you, on the word of a prince, they shall be duly paid you." QUEEN OF ENGLAND *to her Soldiers*, 1588.

WITH THREE ILLUSTRATIVE DIAGRAMS.

LONDON
SMITH, ELDER, & CO. 65 CORNHILL.
1859

PREFACE.

This book is not a work of invention. It is no fancy-piece, but "an ower true tale," as it would be easy to show. The materials are for the most part contained in the Reports of various Commissions, and in the Evidence on which those Reports are based; and the largest amount has been supplied by the latest authorities,—especially the Report and Evidence on the Sanitary Condition of the Army, communicated last year.

The Statistical Statements are illustrated by three diagrams showing the Sanitary State of the Army during the War in the Crimea, for permission to use which I am indebted to the Publishers of "A Contribution to the Sanitary History of the British Army," in which they originally appeared.

It cannot be necessary to explain at any length the inducements to prepare this volume. We sustained a fearful misfortune in the last war: we were taught by a duplicate experience the causes of the loss of our soldiers, and the means of preserving our forces in future: the war has been over nearly three years: there has been no sufficient reason for any it may suffice to rouse the public to claim the complete fulfilment of the programme of reform, laid down by the Royal Commissioners, approved by the authorities at the War-Office, and assented to by all rational persons who have considered the particulars.

There is now a general expectation of war in Europe: and when there is war in Europe, each nation must stand on its defence. We have lavished life, means, and hard money, for very poor results, as regards the maintenance of an adequate military force. We now see how we may maintain an adequate military force at a much smaller cost in every way; and to do this, all that is necessary is such a vigorous expression of the national will as may overcome the obscure resistance in official quarters which always impedes reform in any department of the State. If this will is exerted in time, our national destinies are secure. If not, we shall slide back into the mismanagement, helplessness, and doomed condition from which the bitter experience of the Crimean war should have roused us beyond relapse. I here offer my small contribution to the national safety in the form of a popular presentment of the case.

For the form and construction of the book, I am, as I have said, responsible. The material I have accounted for. I need only say further that the correctness of the technicalities has been secured by the revisal of one whose knowledge on such points makes all safe. Except in regard to these technical expressions, the responsibility of the work as a book is wholly my own.

I believe the story it contains to be altogether true. I believe the inferences and suggestions of the Royal Commissioners to be of vital importance to our national welfare. Thus believing, I could not but offer the facts, inferences, and suggestions in the most popular form in which I could invest them, hoping that they would work strongly on the national judgment and will.

It has been a grave work,—too stern to admit of the indulgence of passionate emotions, such as swept like a torrent over the national heart when the calamity was at its height. In such a story as this there are many incitements to grief, indignation, shame, and compassion, pride, admiration, even hero and heroine worship; but the substantial character of the material, and the gravity and urgency of the use to be made of it, have been an admonition to me to repress all weakening emotions, to avoid both censure and praise, and to be as impersonal as possible, in regard both to myself and to those whom, in their efforts to save our national armies, I would honour and serve.

The Knoll, Ambleside:
April 9th, 1859.

CONTENTS.

CHAPTER I.

LOST ARMIES.

CHAP. II.

PRESERVATION HENCEFORTH—DESTRUCTION HITHERTO.

CHAP. III.

GOING OUT TO WAR.

CHAP. IV.

MEETING THE ENEMY.

CHAP. V.

A WINTER IN CAMP.

CHAP. VI.

PHYSICIANS, IN HEALTH AND DISEASE.

CHAP. VII.

THE WOUNDED AND SICK.

CHAP. VIII.

RESTORATION.

CHAP. IX.

WHAT REMAINS?

ILLUSTRATIONS.

ENGLAND AND HER SOLDIERS.

CHAPTER I.

LOST ARMIES.

Loss by Accident. — HERE and there in history occurs the total loss of an army; and nothing in history makes a stronger impression on young and old. The best-remembered passage in Herodotus is apparently that little paragraph * which relates to the fate of Cambyses' army, sent against the people of Ammon. It is only a few lines: — The army of the Persians was said to have reached a certain spot, but no one could verify the fact. All that was certain was, that it did not reach Ammon, and that it never returned to Egypt. Some reported that, while the troops were taking a meal in the desert, a strong south wind overwhelmed them with mountains of sand, — "and thus perished this army." The image

* Herod. Book III. xxvi.

of this vast, instantaneous death and burial in the heart of the desert has haunted men's imagination for two thousand years. The hot sands are not more striking than the snows. Snowdrifts have overwhelmed armies from the days when Central Asia was advanced in civilisation till now, when the people have to trust to the elements for a defence against the Russians. For generations to come there will be a vivid image in men's minds of the Russian expedition to Khiva in 1839, the greater part of the troops never having returned. The thirty thousand men, with their imposing artillery, waiting for weeks on the bleak steppe before they could embark on the inland sea; their constant successes in skirmishes after landing from the Aral Lake; the muffling of the thunder of their guns by the relentless fall of the snow; the burial of thousands of the living and the dead in the drifts; and the wild desperation of the few who found their way back: these facts make up some of the imagery of our century, which will not be forgotten. So it will be with our own calamity in the Affghanistan war, whence the enemy vowed that only one man should return, and whence only one man did return to bring the first news, though more were soon recovered. So it will be in France with regard to the expedition in Algeria lost above twenty years ago from snow-storm, in a region where it had not been anticipated. Such a conquest of conquerors by such a quiet agency as that of soft-falling snow and drifting sand, is too striking to the imagination ever to die out of the memory.

Loss by Disease. — More armies have, however, been lost by disease than by any kind of sudden accident, or by ill-fortune in warfare. The disease which cuts off thousands of every soldiery sent out to the wars has been heretofore considered more in the light of a natural incident than the bloodshed of warfare on the one hand, and the vengeance of the elements on the other: and this is probably the reason why nations made no progress for centuries in guarding against this kind of mortality. The Czar would not a second time send an expedition to Khiva in the same season, and by the same route; and no English or French commander would evacuate Caubul in midwinter, or expose a force in an African wilderness in weather more formidable than Abd-el-Kader and all his Arabs. But there is not even this degree of prudence in regard to the fatality of disease. The calamity happens almost as often as war itself; and with a sameness of circumstance which ought, in itself, to have been a sufficient warning. Cambyses, sending out an expedition from Thebes against the Ethiopians with a deficient commissariat, witnessed some things very like what have been seen in modern times: — the endurance of hunger at first, — the dropping behind to die, — the eating the beasts of burden and the weeds and shrubs by the wayside; and the difficulty at length what to do with the dead bodies, till turning back was the only thing left to do. The cannibalism (if true) is almost the only feature which has not its representation in the retreat of the French from Moscow; — a disaster which finds its place here, rather than among the accidents from weather, because the army was destroyed by disease and want to a much greater degree than by frost and snow. In all ages, troops have died off "like flies" in marshes; and yet armies still perish in the same way. For a practical purpose, let us just glance at the experience we British have had since the opening of the present century, and at the use we have made of it; and at the reasons for supposing that we have arrived at a turning point in that kind of experience and conduct.

Walcheren.—It is just half a century since we lost an army at Walcheren. We are apt to suppose it much more, because the amount of indignation, grief, and shame spent upon it have been enough for a great calamity, overshadowing a remote age. But it happened within the memory of some of us. The sons of Mr. Wilberforce may possibly remember the spectacle, if they were by his side, on the Sussex cliffs, when he saw the great armament sailing by. He was full of misgivings; and he probably expressed them at the moment, as he did in letters the same day. There were 245 vessels of war and transports, which carried 40,000 troops,—a larger British force than Marlborough ever had under his command; and many thousands of them were under doom,—to die, as men said in those times, "by the visitation of God," but, as is now beginning to be understood, by the murderous ignorance and folly of man.

A book had been published long before by Sir John Pringle, surgeon-general to our forces in Zealand, in which particulars were given of the sickness and death of some of our soldiery, who were stationed sixty years before in Walcheren and a neighbouring island, the narrative clearly marking the limits of the sickly season. Yet the expedition of 1809 sailed without the means of getting over the ground quickly, without maps, and with only one guide, in the very month of July which was pointed out as the first of the sickly season, with only one hospital-ship (though entreaties had been urged for more), and with a wholly insufficient store of medicines and comforts for the sick. There was one person at least who could have told the ministers what must become of a soldiery left on the island of Walcheren in August. Sir Lucas Pepys was aware that Walcheren was the worst place for marsh fever in the known world, except Batavia. He was President of the Medical Board; but he was not consulted till six weeks after the sailing of the expedition. In their anxiety to conceal the destination of the force, Ministers sacrificed the force itself. If they had let the medical officers of the army into their secret, there would at least have been bark on board,—which plain precaution was neglected.

By the middle of August, 3000 men were down in the fever. It must be owing, said their officers, to the stench from the dead bodies of the enemy, which were not buried deep enough in the sand. The sand too was wet and slimy with the ooze of the canals. The waters rose, flooded the British lines, and put out the fires; and the men had to stand in the water and sleep on damp ground. Several thousands of them were up to the waist in water for a whole night. On board the hospital-ship they did not revive. The water they drank was alive with insects; and so were the intestines of the unhappy patients: the nausea and vomiting could not be surmounted. Of the seasoned inhabitants, one-third were ill every season, in spite of high feeding, constant smoking, and other precautions; but the supplies of our troops were short, and nothing could be obtained except from home. Lord Chatham did not see that he could do anything more when the men were dropping at the rate of 200 a day; and he set sail for England on the 14th of September, leaving 8000 men on the sick list. The week before, he had proposed to Government the erection of barracks and other works, at an expense of 100,000*l.*,—his coadjutor, Sir Eyre Coote, writing on the same day that the case was desperate, in a military view, and that the inhabitants of Walcheren, in addition to our own forces, must be fed from England, if the island was to be retained. On the 29th of September, he wrote that three weeks more of the fever would destroy every chance, unless he were immediately reinforced. By the 6th of October he could undertake for nothing more; and by the 22nd he had only 4000 men fit for duty. On the 27th he gave notice that the sick must be abandoned in case of any attack from the enemy,—29,000 of whom were lying close at hand. What were Ministers doing during these dreary weeks?

On the 2nd of September, Lord Castlereagh received the hospital report, which told the state of things, and desired immediate aid in the shape of bark and wine, and other medical comforts, and also of doctors. It took Ministers three weeks to send off one staff-surgeon and five nurses,—without either wine or bark. The doctors were by that time down in the fever; and the healthy men were not enough to attend to the sick. Instead of wine and bark, the Government had sent over water, at the rate of 500 tons a week. The commander and the medical officers did not see what they could do with it; and it was distributed to the fleet. Workmen were sent over, to mend the roofs which had let in the night dews, and to provide means (in the absence of sufficient bedding) to raise the poor fellows from the damp ground; but the workmen took the fever, and made matters worse.

Ministers now took the alarm, and ordered off to Walcheren all the chief officers of the medical department of the army. Each one of these officers tried to shift the duty upon another. The War-office decided that Sir Lucas Pepys, the Physician-General, was the proper person to go,—duly accompanied; but the old gentleman declared that he knew nothing of the investigation of camp and contagious diseases; that his going would be a mere form; and that others, whom he named, were more fit for the errand than an infirm man of nearly seventy, like himself. Even in those days, this was a little too bad; he and the Surgeon-General were dismissed from their posts; and a new Medical Department was established. Happily for the troops, there were some better men than these at their service, though able to do little for them. Instead of removing the force to a healthier site, or merely shifting them out of the slime upon the living waters, or the dry sand-hills, the authorities took time to make up their minds, and compose their quarrels, about evacuating the island; and meanwhile 2000 men died, and 12,000 fell sick. Sir Eyre Coote resigned at the end of October, and was succeeded by General Don, who carried away the last remnant of our force on the 23rd of December.

Some of the statistics of this case remain, though the medical records are lost: and it is wonderful that the known facts have not proved more instructive than they have been. Of the force, which was larger than any British force under Marlborough, 12,863 were sent to England sick in ninety-seven days; and in five months from the next New Year's Day the number of the Walcheren soldiery admitted into the hospitals at home was no less than 36,500.

The Peninsular War. — Before following the Walcheren convalescents into their next adventure, we find ourselves looking about for evidences of the kind of instruction derived from the wretched experience of the Scheldt expedition. One such chapter of calamity was surely enough; and the lesson need never be repeated. So any observer would say.

It was far otherwise. There was plenty of censure, no doubt. Ministers, generals, doctors, were all blamed in proportion to the damage done: but no advance seems to have been made towards keeping the troops healthy next time.

That next time was immediately, — in the early part of the Peninsular war. When Wellington wanted food for his troops, there was no getting money from home, though Ministers were supplying the wants of our allies on the continent by commodities in kind, furnished by contractors who were growing rapidly rich on the war prices thus created. When Wellington employed his own credit to the utmost, and organised the most politic schemes for obtaining flour and rice from America, Ministers provoked a war with the United States. By obtaining the neutrality of Portugal, and freedom from capture for vessels in Portuguese waters, he secured food enough to prevent the war coming to a disastrous close; but no skill, caution, or perseverance of his could preserve his soldiery from the effect of precarious and insufficient food. They ate acorns, or made two rations last for two days, or fell behind from sheer hunger many a time when every man was wanted. The Government which left it mainly to the general to feed his army, could not take the same liberty about the clothing. Coats, head-gear, and shoes do not grow in the fields, and must be sent from home: and the management was of a piece with all the rest. After a march knee-deep in puddled clay, in which the men lost their shoes, they might be barefoot, and therefore stationary during precious days and weeks; and when the shoes did arrive, the probability was that they would be unwearable. It will be remembered that a critical expedition was spoiled by the entire supply of shoes, long waited for, being found too small. The rationale of shelter was not then understood: and the experience of Walcheren was not perhaps imparted in the Peninsula. Everybody knew that lying on wet ground was unwholesome; but the mischief of crowding, and even of bad smells, was not appreciated. Fever and contagion,—contagion and fever,—we read of from 1809 to 1814, though with ups and downs which ought to have been more instructive to us than they were.

In the valley of the Guardiana, in 1809, the Walcheren practices were forestalled, and the same consequences ensued. The troops were well fed at the moment, from Badajoz: but they were set down on the wet sands of the valley; 7,000 were in hospital at once, and nearly two-thirds of them died. Wellington could then produce only 25,000 men, in face of the French 90,000. He weathered that year; but the nation asked how he was to get through the next, with a force so extensively and frequently *hors de combat.*

The sick were throughout a heavy burden,—more than enough to occupy one man's wits; and yet it did not strike anybody that the Commander-in-Chief ought to have been relieved of that charge. To the Medical Department the sick were a far heavier charge than the wounded; and yet nobody took the hint to preclude the difficulty, by confining the sickness within the narrowest possible limits. During the entire Peninsular war, the average sickness was 21 in 100 of the soldiery. Considering the costliness, as well as uselessness, of every sick soldier, the delays he imposed, the burden he was, the attendance he required, it seems as if the sickness was the great affliction of the whole war. And so it was; the killed and wounded were a very small number in comparison. That a fifth part of the force was laid prostrate, occupying the time and strength of hundreds or thousands who could ill be spared, was the most wearing of Wellington's cares, and the most calamitous incident of the war.

Who, what, and where were these sick? The largest proportion of them were the Walcheren convalescents, who had been sent from the hospitals at home, assured, probably, that the voyage would complete the restoration of their strength, but who sank under the first hot noon or dewy night. Wherever they were dispersed, down they sank, whenever the causes of fever were present; and there were few halting places exempt from those causes. Next to the Walcheren men, the new levies, or fresh importations, suffered most; and thirdly, the Peninsular convalescents. These were the sick. As for what their diseases were, fever was, as has been said, constant and supreme. Inflammation of the lungs, rheumatism, sore-throat, and catarrh were all prevalent; and the scourge of hospital gangrene and lock-jaw, was sure to appear in every assemblage of the wounded. We read of dismal appearances of prostration: of yellow skin, cold and inert; of livid eruptions, and constant tendenoy to mortification; and, as a matter of course, of an extraordinary disproportion of dead to sick. As to where these poor wretches were laid down, when they could not hold up their heads, it is, perhaps, the most important of the questions concerned.

The medical authorities could not deal with their patients without hospitals; and yet, sending them to hospital was usually sending them to death. No casual shelter, provided from point to point, could afford means of attendance and treatment to the sick and wounded. They must be concentrated, in order to be attended to; yet, as often as they were collected, fever set in, and gangrene made a more rapid sweep of the wounded. There were hospitals all along the roads of march; and they were dismal places, — indispensable but hopeless. It was not negligence; everything was attempted that the doctors could ask or the commander provide. From bleeding to cayenne pepper, it has been said, everything was tried; but nothing availed. It was knowledge that was wanted; and, if the knowledge was not ready on demand, teachableness. Whenever, in reading the histories of that war, we find the troops in an improved condition, we perceive that they have had not only food, rest, clothes and blankets, but active business in the open air. Towards the end of the war we obtain, by putting this and that together, some striking hints about economising an army. The Guards, it may be remembered, were *hors de combat* for above half a year, from November 1812 to June 1813, from fever; and the whole army had been so often depressed by the burden of illness, that large numbers had got into the habit of "skulking." Six hundred bayonets in one month, Napier's

History tells us, were recovered to the second division alone, by clearing the hospitals and depôts of malingerers before the battle of Vittoria. After that battle, the Guards rejoined the army, every available man of the force was busy in the open air of the mountains, fortifying passes, and going to and from the coast for supplies; and, though the snow was deep, the weather severe at times, and the nights cold, the troops enjoyed such health as they had not known since they entered the country. Those who were sent by sea, in crowded and dirty transports, to any of the stations below, became hospital subjects immediately; while their comrades in the Pyrenees, harassed by long marches and cold vigils, showed the lowest rate of mortality. The Guards were taken special care of, being quartered in towns and villages; but they were prostrated by fever, dysentery, and the whole tribe of diseases which their comrades in the open air had escaped. Such was the state of things in the winter of 1813–1814, when the officials at home had not sent out even the great coats for the soldiers. Money was excessively scarce; the food which was landed at Santander was detained, from the Spanish authorities having placed the British hospitals there in quarantine, and discredited Santander everywhere; and under these disadvantageous circumstances, the force descended to the wet lowlands on the French side, at a critical season. On the morning before the final battle of Toulouse, the sick of the British force, present and absent, were a little short of 13,000, out of a total of 56,000. During the Peninsular war, a number nearly equal to our whole force passed through the hospitals twice every year. The deaths were 18,500; and adding to these the 4500 returned to England incapacitated, we have 23,000 men lost as soldiers. When we consider, in addition, the loss, delay, damage, and suffering occasioned by the 324,672 cases which passed through the hospitals to renewed service, we shall think it strange that we did not profit by such a lesson, sufficiently at least to lose no more armies from sickness. Yet we have since lost armies from that set of causes; and have, from our small kingdom, supplied 164 soldiers for every effective 100, when, by having learned from experience, we might have done better with 105. Even this is classing the attendants on the sick with the effectives. A waste, as to mere numbers, of 50 to every 100 men is no small matter to a nation the size of ours. But this is forestalling what can be said to more advantage afterwards.

First Birman War. — It would seem difficult to throw away an army by sickness between the beginning and the end of our forty years' peace. Yet we achieved something like it in 1824 and 1825, in our invasion of the Birman Empire. The details show that Lord Amherst and his officials had not studied the Walcheren and the Peninsular cases to any great purpose. When Sir

Thomas Munro, then governor of Madras, heard of the inconvenience caused by the encroachments of the Birmese in Chittagong in. 1823, he concluded that the mischief would be met on the spot, and dealt with, as such difficulties may usually be, by patience in asserting the true superiority of force, at convenient seasons. When drawn upon for troops, he lent his last sepoy,— wondering at the policy which rushed forward to encounter destruction in the swamps of Ava, but concluding that a dashing campaign was intended,— such as would be most imposing to a barbaric enemy, and soonest over. When he perceived that the responsible parties went to work as Marlborough might for a German campaign,— with everything ponderous and slow,— he foresaw what must happen. Yet others knew as well as he that the country which the army was to traverse was a great alluvion, where the inhabitants built their houses on piles, and wild beasts were driven to the highest part of the jungles by floods. Others must have known as well as he the importance of some survey of the *terrain* before carrying the troops into the malaria; of obtaining some knowledge of the routes and passes, the floodings and shoalings of the great rivers, and the probabilities of getting on, and of obtaining the means of conveyance and subsistence. These points ascertained, the passage up the country might either be delayed till the best season, or effected with speed.

Sir Thomas Munro said that such a method "would have saved much time,"— meaning that it would have saved much life. As it was, he regarded the expedition as a "romantic and visionary" enterprise; and the results long appeared visionary enough.

When our troops were sinking under sun-stroke, fever, and dysentery in swamp and jungle, it was no comfort that the Birmese suffered more, for they did not make peace. They ran away at every opportunity, and left their ammunition and the corpses of their dead to us; and our soldiers sat in the reeking marsh, with tropical rains pouring down on them, dying the faster for there being no foe within reach to rouse their energies. One-eighth were soon sick; and then the enemy returned, and fired upon them from the jungles. Every delay afforded further opportunity to the natives to destroy their magazines and lay waste their fields; so that when Sir Archibald Campbell and his haggard soldiery at length reached Rangoon, they found themselves in danger of starving. There was nothing to be done but to obtain provisions by the river from its mouth; and the perpetual transit through the malarious regions was always adding to the sum of mortality. It was not till February 1826 that peace was made; and whatever else lingered and procrastinated, disease and death did not. What the mortality really was perhaps nobody knows; it might have been prudent to let it pass.

Second Birman War.—If other lessons did not take effect, one would think that a deadly war in Birmah would be a caution against a second deadly war in Birmah. But even this was too much to expect, so lately as within ten years. General Godwin reached the mouth of the Irawaddy on the 2nd of April, 1852; and at the end of the year, when complaint was made that nothing was gained, the answer was the old one,—tropical rains, tropical suns, swamps, jungles, no roads;—no facilities for warfare, as soldiers understand it, and death lying in wait at every step. It was not till the middle of 1853 that peace was made, and by the time we heard of it the interest of the Russian controversy was at its height. Even that conflict, and the fearful watch we had to keep upon the Crimea, have not effaced the impression of the calamities in Birmah. The news of cholera and dysentery that came by every ship from India, the slowness of General Godwin, and the melancholy excuses for that slowness, we cannot have forgotten. They showed that we had not yet learned how to protect and economise an army.

Before contemplating the yet more signal proof of this apparent perverseness afforded by the Russian war, and by every party engaged in it, it will be well to consider, with some precision, what it was that we had to learn. This being ascertained, we shall perceive what reason there is to hope that the instruction is really obtainable, and that we have obtained it.

CHAP. II.

PRESERVATION HENCEFORTH.—DESTRUCTION HITHERTO.

WHAT was the lesson, precisely, that we had to learn?

What is wanted.—In a superficial way, the answer seems easy enongh:—not to lodge an army in a swamp;—not to send them out on service in a tropical noon, nor to choose the rainy season for a campaign;—not to stifle them, nor starve them, nor freeze them, nor scorch them. But these are the answers which might and would have been given before our Walcheren, and Peninsular, and Birman disasters, as fluently as now. The ideas they contain are true; but, as answers, they are inappropriate and barren. They give an instance for a principle,—like the Sunday scholar, who, being asked what hypocrisy was, replied "Pretending to walk lame." They are barren, because a mere list of unwholesome conditions, apart from principles and organisation, can never put into the hands of any commander the means of preserving the health of his army.

Who is responsible.—The Commander has always

supposed the Doctors undertook the health of the force: and it does not appear that at home the Medical Department of the army has thought of disputing the assignment. But when it comes to service abroad, a difficulty arises; the physicians see that mischief must come of encamping in some particular spot, or exercising under certain conditions: but the military officers say it is necessary, and cannot be helped; and thus the soldiers are doomed. But, if the case is no better at home, — if the soldiers die faster than other people in their own climate and their own barracks, — is not that the fault of the physicians?

Why, no. And here we are again reminded of the lesson we had to learn through the repeated loss of armies. The physicians could not have saved the Walcheren force from fever, nor the Peninsular army from dysentery and rheumatism. Their business was to treat sick and wounded men; and not to preserve the health of the healthy. My readers may possibly start at this; but a very little consideration will show them that it is true. The physician and surgeon profess to understand, and to be able to treat, diseased and injured human frames. This is their proper business; and it is quite enough. It is a special study, — that of the diseased or injured human body; and, like every special study and art, it requires the whole mind of the student and practitioner. But it is also true, that the study of hygiene, which is not only different from those of medicine and surgery, but of an opposite character, requires a different, if not an opposite, kind of mind from that which makes a good physician. If there is any hesitation about assenting to this, it must be because the nature of hygienic study and practice is not accurately understood; and the absence of this understanding is a fresh evidence that the physician has not been a hygienic resource hitherto, or he would have been an exponent of the science, and a practitioner of the art, as a matter of course. He would have saved our armies:—a thing which no physician, or Medical Department, ever did yet, or could reasonably be expected to do.

Have our physicians at home saved our poor townspeople from fever and cholera? Have we even now physicians qualified by training and experience to undertake the charge of keeping our population healthy? We have not. The civil officers of health may be physicians; but our physicians have never been trained to be officers of health. They caution individual patients against what is bad for them—as we say, "put their case into their own hands;" but, when the question is of instituting such conditions as shall promote and protect the health of a whole society, physicians are not prepared with either principles, facts, or methods. The most enlightened civil officers of health are the most aware of the very small progress yet made in either the science or the art of hygiene; and the best results of their inquiries that we are yet in possession of, are of a merely provisional character, because the very bases of classification on which their estimates are founded must be held subject to correction and change. The whole inquiry is so modern, the conditions of the bodily welfare of a complicated population are so far from being settled, in a scientific sense, and the nomenclature of maladies depends so essentially on those ill-understood conditions, that the most orderly-looking tables and averages must be received as material which remains to be tested, and which is certain to be more or less wrong. Till, for instance, the whole world of sanitary science is agreed as to the proper quantity of fresh air for every individual, as to the chemical history of all main articles of diet, and as to the contagion and infection questions, there can be no trustworthy classification of maladies, or permanent nomenclature, such as is indispensable for sanitary statistics.

Hygiene.—The science and art of hygiene having become manifest in modern times, the lesson we could not learn before, and must learn now, is its application to the preservation of our armies, at home and abroad. We have found that, even amidst our scanty knowledge and small skill in sanitary affairs, life and health may be saved with such certainty, and in such clear proportions, that carelessness in regard to conditions is fast assuming its proper character of moral and social offence: and the natural impulse is to apply our new knowledge and powers to the army, as that aggregate of our population—that department of the nation—which has recently exhibited the most fearful amount of mortality on record in the history of centuries.

As soon as this application is attempted, the truth appears that another distinction has to be attended to. This is quite in the natural course of things. The advance of science is always marked by the disclosure of new distinctions and differences. Some of us can remember the time when Chemistry was spoken of as a single branch of knowledge; and now it has already unfolded itself into a vast and diversified region of inquiry, containing so many departments that the best minds can obtain only a mere glance of the whole, and are quite satisfied each to work in one. In somewhat the same way, men used to suppose everything connected with the human body to be one subject: but anatomy was soon seen to be one thing and physiology another, and the surgical art to be wholly different from the medical. While awaiting the further divisions which experience and analogy teach us to expect, we find we have been confounding the protection of health with the treatment of disease; and, yet again, that Civil and Military Hygiene are different things in the practical sense in which the unprofessional world is concerned with them.

Civil and Military Hygiene.— The Commissioners who have reported on the sanitary affairs of the army give us their description of Military Hygiene. They say, "It is sanitary science applied to the prevention of disease and mortality under conditions far more varied, more threatening to health, and, above all, more sudden and novel in their character, than those which affect the health of men engaged in the ordinary avocations of life." Thus, Military Hygiene is the sanitary science of the world generally, with additions required by the peculiarities of the military condition. Whatever is true and right about supplies of pure air and pure water in a town, is true and right in a camp: damp and bad smells are offences everywhere; cleanliness and bodily exercise are everywhere essential to health. So far, and a good deal farther, Civil and Military Hygiene may march together. But the sanitary science requisite for keeping in health an army during a course of foreign service,—and even in barracks at home,—is special, and must be provided for accordingly. This is so obvious, that I need not illustrate it at any length. One set of sanitary officers, the civil, has to attend to streets full of houses, supplied with an apparatus of drains, good, bad, or indifferent; and another, the military, if it existed, would have to deal with an area which might have been a heath the day before, or a swamp, or a village green,—it may be a valley or a table-land, a hollow or a slope.

The civil sanitary officer has always a river or other water-supply at hand, flowing in permanent channels: military officers of health would have to look after the water-supply in every new place. At home, the people spontaneously dress according to the seasons, and the climate is a matter of course; whereas in foreign warfare, our soldiers have various risks to run from heat and cold; and, thus far, their clothing has not been particularly adapted to circumstances. At home, our fellow-citizens buy their food as they like; and the supply of all essentials in the market is as steady as if it were regulated by a law of nature, as in fact it is; whereas an army has to be fed by a department organised for the purpose, and in an artificial way. While in London the daily supply of milk comes to every door, as punctual as the air and the light, in the camp every item of every man's food is bought, and fetched, and delivered by a series of acts of forethought and management. These are specimens of the differences of the two modes of life, in regard to sanitary care. But it is also true that the difference extends from the conditions into the results of health and disease. There are diseases to which soldiers, and others to which civilians, are particularly liable. Army physicians are, therefore, not the best advisers in medical practice at home; and civil officers of health would not be equal to the sanitary duties of the army. The mode of life at home is natural (to the individuals, though not in the final philosophical sense); whereas the life of warfare, — of modern warfare, — is artificial in a high degree. While, therefore, the function of the sanitary officer is special, because hygiene is a newly-discovered branch of knowledge, the function of the military hygienic officer is doubly special, — a special function founded on a special division of knowledge.

This is the lesson we have now to learn,—not only as we know it at present, as an idea, but as a practical truth. After having lost an army at the outset of every war we have engaged in, we have at last enjoyed the blessing of seeing one saved. It was this which was wanted to enable us to take home the lessons of experience. We have witnessed and endured a more appalling loss than any former one: we have witnessed the restoration of a perishing force to the highest condition of health and efficiency ever known; and from the double illustration we have learned what to aim at, and to do, in order to preserve the British army, and provide, in the wisest manner, for the military defence of the empire. We have ascertained that the wisest way of doing this is precisely that which is most economical of life, most conservative of health, and least burdensome to the national finances.

Another consideration is sufficiently obvious. We are declared to be not a military nation, by taste or destiny,—not able, except by our wealth, to compete in national strength with continental states, which, having a wider area, and a larger population, can supply larger armies, and support a severer drain. There is no occasion to discuss the points of taste and destiny here. The practical consideration is, how far the preservation of our soldiers is equivalent to a larger power of supply. If we were to go on losing, by disease, sixty-four soldiers to every hundred effective ones, while other nations were suffering in the same way in their armies, war would become difficult to us within a period easily assignable; but, if we can keep up the excellence of vigour attained by us in the Crimea, before the close of the war, and have to manage only five sick to every hundred of effective soldiers, while other armies, behind us in hygienic science and skill, are sinking in "pestilence," "dying like flies," going through, in short, what we have endured, we shall hold a very secure position in regard to military power and consideration. We none of us doubt, probably, that England's arm can keep her head; but it will mark a new period in our honour and welfare, when we can prove that the military profession is, with us, little, if at all, more perilous than various civil occupations. The positive increase to our strength and prestige could not but be great, from the moment the fact was established; and upon this would follow an improvement in the prime material of our military force. The recruits in a doomed or suffering army will, for the most part, be men who can do no better for themselves — incapable or reckless. Substitute safety from degrading discomfort and disease for the life and death of a dog in a ditch, and our actual army will be in future what the poet has dreamed that it was, and the patriot demands, and the statesman resolves that it shall be.

The Life of the Soldier.—What has the soldier's life been hitherto, before the discovery of the way to take care of it? During our forty years' peace, there was no room for romancing about the perils of the field, the awful chances of the siege, and the shedding of blood in the service of the country. What was it, then, which made the Queen's service so fatal, and which was for ever pulling down the best strength of the army, and dooming our defenders to more danger and death than they had expected, without any of the glory?

In order to see how it was, let us glance at the way of living of the men before they were soldiers, and at that of their acquaintance who are not soldiers.

The Material.—I have in my mind's eye a small country town, of about 2000 inhabitants. It is a quiet, old-fashioned place, very well satisfied with itself, very dull (which it takes for gentility), and yet exceedingly proud if anybody born in it makes any noise in the world. In fact, it is shocked and offended, and rather cruel, if any inhabitant broaches a new idea; but it makes up for the cruelty at last, by being delighted and adulatory when that fame is reflected back upon it which sprang out of the very ideas so shocking when they were new. One of its characteristic inhabitants was an old lady, who scolded a young lady for asking a subscription to a school for girls; the old lady not wanting to hear anything about educating poor people, as she had had three bad housemaids in succession, all of whom could read and write. One of its characteristic excitements is the poaching-frays, which happen almost every winter. Before and just after Christmas, the signs and tokens appear. The gamekeepers look solemn, and patrol the plantations. The labourers are absent now and then for a day—gone to the county town—unless the carrier brings a message from the poulterer, and effects a mysterious meeting in the highroad by starlight, to receive certain sacks, out of which feathers or fur may be peeping. There is a savoury smell about some of the poor cottages—not exactly what might be expected from dinners of potatoes and buttermilk, nor even of bacon and greens; and when the housewife says she fears her children will have only a crust for their Christmas-dinner, she is complimented on their looks—ruddy as they are when clean. She replies that "they thrive in the dirt." Wages are only eight shillings a week; and there is a debt at the shop, of course. There is more than one shop, however. There is a genteel one, where the business of draper is carried on at one counter, and that of mercer at the other, while there is millinery upstairs. It has not much custom, but what it has is a paying custom; which is far from being the case with the general shop, where the labouring people go for everything they want, and where, at most, two-thirds of the customers pay anything, except on stringent occasions, and where few customers pay more than two-thirds of what they owe. There is a market once a week, and a fair once a year. There is a great law firm, which has all the land business for many miles round; and there is a brewery; and there is a bank—in a room which can admit two customers before the desk and counter, and the banker and his clerk behind them.

On a fair-day, and on more than one market-day, the lively presence of the recruiting-sergeant has spread excitement through the town. From the great farms in the neighbourhood he has gleaned five or six young men who will serve the Queen. Thereupon ensues the well-known lament with which the news of an enlistment has always been received there; for, as I have said, it is an old-fashioned place. The curate checks the grief, and so does the squire; but the farmers say it is hard that the strongest young fellows should be drawn off the land. The squire gives in *his* way to the service of his country; and he is of opinion that poor men should be glad to give their personal service. The curate cannot understand where the hardship lies. The youths are going of their own accord; they are quitting a precarious for a certain maintenance; they will have warm house-room, plentiful food, and meat every day; their uniform, certainly much finer than any clothes they ever wore before; their pay, and finally their pension; and, above all, an honourable and patriotic calling, without danger from shot and bayonet, unless war should break out. Even then, while the honour would be higher, the risks would be nothing like what is usually supposed. So says the curate. He observes that it is very natural that in our gratitude to our soldiers in war time, we should dwell much on their sacrifices. A man who returns with only one arm or leg creates a sensation in and beyond his village, which puts out of sight the comrades who have taken no harm. For one soldier who is buried on the battle-field, or who comes back maimed, there are thousands who never were wounded, or who have recovered entirely. The curate really cannot pity a stout young man, who is selected for his bodily advantages; and who, for very easy duty, is to have, without any trouble on his own part, all the main comforts of life daily provided while he is on duty, a doctor and a hospital at hand if he should be ill, and a pension, and some social consideration awaiting him at the close of his active term.

The curate's view prevails with most people; and some ask whether the recruits are not better off than the youth at the bank, who is going to be a clerk in

London, or the draper's second son, who is to be a shopman in Whitechapel. Last week, it was considered a great thing for the two brothers who got precarious employment, with some personal danger, as watchers at the Grange plantations, to obtain appointments in the police of the county-town; but the glory paled before that of the Queen's service.

The glory increases when it appears, as it soon does, that it is not every young man who can serve the Queen, however willing he may be. One or two weakly or deformed youths perhaps looked on with envy at the time of the enlistment. They had no chance, they knew; but now, three out of six who enlisted are sent home again. They did not know that anything ailed them; but their health and strength are not of the prime quality necessary for the military service; and here the farmers renew their complaints, saying that it is very hard upon them, — the best labourers are taken, and the weakly ones are thrown back upon the land.

The City Clerk.—Before a very long time, it becomes apparent that all the youths who hoped great things from going out into the world must pay a pretty heavy tax in health for whatever advantages they obtain. The young clerk looks worse and worse, each time that he pays a visit home. He lives in a city lodging, and has a dead wall opposite his chamber window, so close that it is only in summer weather that he can see to dress. He is stooping over his desk all day, except Sundays; and he spends his evenings in reading, or in occasional visits to friends, or to the theatres. He seldom sees a hedge or a pond, or a common, except in his annual week at home, when the fresh air and the light are almost too much for his weakened head. He grows yellower, and pines more, as his salary rises; and when his father learns from a medical friend that the city clerk's occupation is considered nearly the most unhealthy of any, he says it will not do; and no son of his shall pay down his life for any post in any merchant's house, which he might occupy only to die.

The Shopman.—The shopman in Whitechapel has not to complain of sitting at a desk all day; for his grievance is standing. The discipline is as severe as that of a regiment. He must be always bolt upright, — leaning neither against the shelves behind, nor the counter before him; talking to nobody but the customers, from seven in the morning till nine at night, with the exception of the short mealtimes, — ten minutes each for breakfast and tea, and a quarter of an hour for dinner. Too tired to stand, and losing the power of brisk walking, the shopman sees as little of the country as the clerk. He sleeps in a dormitory with forty or fifty of his comrades,—their beds two feet apart, and the windows so few as to leave the place always dim, and in the morning hot and close. When the young shopman runs home for a holiday, he lolls on the sofa, sleeps late, cannot trouble himself to go round and see the old places, and complains to the doctor of an aching back and swollen legs.

The diet is noble at his employer's;—legs of prime mutton, surloins, beefsteaks, the best vegetables and bread, the meals served hot, the large urns of coffee and tea steaming as fragrant as in any West-end *restaurant:* but though the strength may be kept up for a time by generous diet, the appetite soon fails. Food that is bolted is mischievous, be its quality what it may: and a digestion weakened by an unnatural course of life benefits less by mutton and vegetables than a vigorous one by bread and water. The shopman's lot is not much better than the clerk's.

The Policeman.—The policemen's ought to be worse, however, the neighbours think. The brothers must find the difference between watching game and patrolling a city. The policeman must be out in all weathers. People in their warm beds hear the rain pelt against their windows while the policeman is out in it. In the dog-days he may be seen squeezing himself into some shady corner at noon-day for a little release from the glare; but he must not sit down, nor stay long enough to grow cool. At midnight he may take shelter in a doorway from a gush of rain, but he must trudge through a steady down-pour till he is relieved. Night-duty for eight months in the year, and exposure, must surely be the worst possible things for health, to say nothing of the risks run by the police among thieves and brawlers. Others remark, on the other side of the case, the regular intervals of rest, the good clothing, the stout cloth coat, the oilskin hat and cape, and the thick boots. They say that the night duty is light,—being chiefly that of watching for eight hours without sitting down. The day duty is far more laborious, and therefore it is divided into two periods of four hours. Is it the night work or the hard work that is complained of? If the first, it is certainly not a natural mode of life: but then it is not laborious, and is relieved by entire rest. If the latter, it is broken up into periods, and those periods combined make up a day's work less hard than thousands of labourers are accustomed to. Then the unmarried policemen have good shelter, warmth, and meals at their quarters; their sleeping-rooms are less crowded than the dormitories of many private establishments, and they are well attended in sickness. Why should the policeman be particularly pitied? "Because they suffer more, and die sooner, than people in general," says the odd gentleman of the town. Every little town has one odd gentleman at least who knows just what nobody else has ever thought of learning, and comes out as an oracle when nobody else has an idea to bestow. "If out of a thousand policemen, with their short terms of service, nearly nine die in every year, while only seven in a thousand die of men of the same age who live more healthily, I say the policeman may be pitied." Thus declares the oracle. He considers it rather unfortunate that, of the young men who have left the place, so many should have gone into unhealthy occupations. He is reminded of the young soldiers. *They* must have changed for the better, surely. The oracle replies that time will show; and after a moment's thought, he observes that it is strange that one seldom sees a private soldier above forty.

The Soldier.—The recruits;—what is it that time is to show about them? They are so alike in their fortunes that one may exhibit the destiny of all who ever went from our little town. Bob had always lived in the same cottage. It was a tidy place when his parents married; but now it is a mere hovel. Those brick cottages are almost worse than the clay tenements of other counties for standing weather. Mossy in one place and black in another, the walls show signs of crumbling in a quarter of a century, instead of standing for a thousand years, like the dwellings of a mountain region. The wet comes in at corners, and the thatch is rotten in places. The bit of window upstairs will not open; but that does not matter, as it is broken, and never mended. It is stopped up with anything that comes to hand: for a man who gets only eight shillings a week cannot employ the glazier. Bob has always slept at the top of the stair, in a nice current of air from the chimney below and the broken window above.

During the day, he has always been abroad in the fields, except when the weather would allow nothing to be done there: and fresh air, bread, bacon, and potatoes have made a stout man of him, though rather round in the shoulders and wabbling in his gait. He has generally carried a pound of good mud on each foot, and never had any nice fancies about the dungheap, three yards from the door. His ruddy face smiled through all the grime; and, as his mother said, he "throve in the dirt." There was a grand prospect before him when he quitted the old home, the mother admitted.

It is true he never thought to live in such a place as the barrack-rooms. He never had such bedding before, nor had seen such, except in the great shop. He had never had beef for dinner every day: and certainly he never before kept his person so clean, nor wore anything like such clothes. Yet his health is not what it always was before. He is perpetually having colds. His coughs return whenever the weather changes. His sleep is disturbed; and he feels ready to hang himself in the morning till the fresh air revives his spirits. He wearies of his meals. He wearies of his drill, and of all his business. He wearies of his very life. When he dreams of the lark in the meadow, he thinks he should like to desert, if he had the spirit; but he knows his lot is cast, and he pines on till some change is appointed him. His chest was expanded at first by the drill; and his walk is soldierly—he even thinks he is grown—but still, he is not the man he was. His health is, in fact, undermined. His clothes are not as good as they are fine. The cloth sucks up wet like a sponge, and thickens and shrinks with it,—having been before like a fine sieve, letting in the cold as easily. His boots burst out before he has worn them a week. He used not to mind the rawest wind on the common; but now he feels the cold whenever he turns out of the warm guard-room into the night air; and if he comes in wet, he must sleep in his damp clothes in a place close with the breath of many comrades. Hence his cough. The first person who enters in the morning says the smell is enough to knock one down. Heavy and head-achy, he must rise and make his bed, and prepare his personal matters, and breakfast at seven. Then there is drill, or guard, as may be; not nearly enough to fill up his day or his thoughts. He is never alone to think in peace; nor can he work with his hands to relieve his dulness. He goes perhaps to new quarters in one place or another, and back again; but there is no prospect of war, or any more enlivening service. If, in addition to these things, he takes a disgust to boiled beef, and if the water is bad to drink, and there are foul smells about from worse causes than the dungheap at home, it is no wonder that he goes into hospital from time to time. In fact, his comrades die off fast,—more than twice as fast as policemen, and nearly three times as fast as the neighbours at home; and it may be expected that poor Bob will perish in consumption, unless he is carried off first by one of those sweeps which fever and cholera make in barracks and other places where the people have not each their portion of fresh air and pure water. It is really true that foot soldiers in barracks at home have died at the rate of above twenty per thousand in a year, while men of the same age, of various ordinary occupations, and in a healthy situation, have died at the rate of only seven in a thousand.

Military Mortality.—As the mortality of barrack life may now be spoken of in the past tense, it is not necessary to dwell on the particulars further than to put them on record. If, as some may think, it is presumptuous to reckon the cessation of the surplus mortality of our soldiers at home, it is at least true that the needed reform has fairly set in. The authorities have their eye on every opportunity of rectifying old evils, and of new lodging the troops under improved sanitary conditions. One way of helping them in accomplishing the work is to keep alive the knowledge of our losses under the old methods, though the time is happily over for complaint and censure. The truth, then, is, that whereas the fine set of young men selected for military service ought to yield a smaller amount of mortality (except under the head of casualties) than any other class, they exhibit a proportion of deaths frightfully large in comparison with the most unhealthy classes of society in general. When the most robust are taken for soldiers, all the inferior candidates are thrown back upon society, to count in the comparison which they render unfair; and again, when the soldier becomes invalided, he is returned upon society in the same way, so that the soldiers are not only "the pick" of mankind in the first instance, but they remain so by transferring to civilian society all who sink below the mark of active duty. If the army had the ordinary chances of health, the soldiers would present the smallest mortality of any class: instead of which we find that twice as many of them die as of the least healthy order of people in Great Britain. The proportion becomes aggravated abroad. Take any set of Englishmen of the same age,—say between 15 and 45,—and you will find the annual mortality 1 in 100 from epidemic and constitutional disease, from local disease, and from violent death collectively; whereas the deaths from those causes were, in our army in the East, nearly 23 per cent.,—only 3 per cent. being from wounds in hospital, while more than 18 were from epidemic disease. The object of introducing this last illustration is to show how little the wounds received in action have to do with the soldier's peril. The deduction of the 3 per cent. for shot, sword, bayonet, and accidents, leaves a mortality of nearly 20 per cent., which is in fact what our finest regiments have exhibited in barracks at home.

This can be no wonder when the horrors of barrack-life,—such as it was till quite recently,—are remembered: the sleeping and eating in the same room, and that room admitting only a pittance of the fresh air necessary for the inmates; the inmates themselves, in their ignorance, stopping up such orifices as did exist; the going in and out on guard at night, when the barrack was hottest and the outer air coldest; the foul smells from ill-placed drains, and from filthy old customs, which, like all customs in public institutions, it was difficult to get changed; the badness and insufficiency of the water in many instances; the monotony of the food; the deficiency of manly exercises; the absence of occupation and interests. Under such an assemblage of unfavourable influences as these, how should men live and be healthy? Consumption and fever have carried them off by tens of thousands, when, by obedience to the clearest of nature's laws, they might have lived to old age.

Before the last war began, when nobody dreamed of soldiers dying faster than farmers or artisans, we now know that in our army, at home and abroad, more than four soldiers died to one man in any healthy district in England. This was during the fifteen years from 1839 to 1853 (inclusive). During that time of peace 58,000 of our soldiers died, of whom 44,500 died to a great extent from mismanagement, and we may say by becoming soldiers, instead of remaining among those who lived and flourished under ordinary influences. The Turk would perhaps make no distinction between unnecessary and unavoidable mortality, between the deaths of forty thousand men in early manhood by fever and consumption, and their departure in a good old age by natural decline; but, unless we are fatalists in the grossest sense, we must regard the sacrifice consummated so lately as 1853 as a national calamity caused by popular ignorance; and every life lost hereafter from the same influences must be considered a case of culpable homicide.

Some persons may be more impressed by the gratuitous mortality in any one year than by even such a result as is yielded by the records of fifteen. If we take any one year, it had better be that in which we are most sure of the numbers all round;—that is the year of the census. In 1851, then, the effective force of the army was 136,277. If these men had lived as ordinary English people of the same time of life do, they would have lost 1,248 by death. If they had lived in the healthiest places, the deaths would have been 1,051. And what was the actual rate of mortality among them, as British soldiers of all arms? Why, 2,381. At that modern date, and in that season of peace, more than twice as many of our soldiers died as if they had remained civilians.

Effect of Reform.—While this was our management, is it any wonder that recruiting was difficult? Is it any wonder that the mental and moral character of our recruits is, or has been, so low? If we want to find where the reckless, the outcast, the idle, the shiftless "most do congregate," it is where there is the chance of "a short life and a merry one." The barrack life of a soldier has, to be sure, not been a very merry one; but it has been the popular notion that it was. Short enough it was, indisputably, to tens of thousands of victims. Now that the tables are turned, and soldiers may, if we choose, have a better chance of health and life than other men, we shall see the difference in the quality of the men who offer for the service. The service will have lost its character of a lottery, where there are many deaths to few rewards. Good treatment, inducing self-respect, raises the character of a soldiery even more than that of other men, inasmuch as honour is theoretically their pursuit. Schools, varied occupation, manly exercise, are all good things, for body and mind; but there are some more essential requisites than even these. Food that will nourish; clothes that will answer the purpose of clothing; cleanliness that will leave nature to work unhindered in each human frame; and a due supply of the most vital element of all,—pure air;—these are the provisions due to the soldier, from the hour of his enlistment. Duly afforded, they will procure us a soldiery worthy of our national name and needs: denied, they will leave our national security to the mercy of the scapegraces and the dolts of society.

The contrast is no fancy-piece. It is no longer necessary to argue by analogy or contrast from the consequences of a bad administration to the anticipated consequences of a good one. The result has been actually worked out. After an army had sunk to the lowest degree of misery and helplessness ever known, short of extinction, it was lifted up into a condition of high health and efficiency, with the lowest rate of mortality on record. The experiment was complete, well defined in all its stages, and recorded for future guidance. As a consequence, we are now in possession of a thorough analysis of the experiment and its conditions; and also of new means of perfecting our experience. We are already lodging, feeding, clothing, occupying, and amusing our soldiers better. We have a camp full of healthy troops at Aldershott, in spite of some unfavourable conditions which would have done deadly mischief among them ten years ago. Thus, it is not being visionary or presumptuous to reckon on a better future for our military strength generally, and a longer and happier life for our soldiers in particular. Nor is it pride to regard our military position among the nations as raised, to a greater degree than it has been lowered within the last ten years. No country could stand the drain of soldiers to which our unreformed methods would have condemned us. Any free country can hold its own, for any length of time, while to the indomitable pluck and endurance of the British soldier is added the self-respect and the comfortable plight of the English citizen.

CHAP. III.

GOING OUT TO WAR.

Hiatus in the War-Scheme.—THE last time war was declared, no arrangement had been made as to who was to have the charge of the health of the army. It was plain enough who was to be responsible for the sick and well; but an utter confusion of ideas existed as to the preservation of health. No doubt it was supposed, in a vague way, as it is in civil life, that health was the natural condition of men, and would take care of itself; whereas the mortality during the seven preceding years of peace was what we have seen. If the question had been asked, how the health of the troops going to the East was provided for,—the answer would have been either that the doctors must see to that, or that the Commissariat would make the men comfortable; whereas the doctors were sure to have their hands full of their own proper business; and the Commissariat could only carry out the articles of necessity and comfort, and had nothing to do beyond supplying them. Was it the military authorities? Did not the Duke of Wellington give his attention to the health of the troops in his wars?—We know the answers. Who was to teach the military authorities about hygiene? And had they not enough to do without entering into the details of the art? The Duke of Wellington did all that a general of his time could do: but the results showed how little that was.

Exploring Commissioners.—But these questions were not asked when we were under the well-remembered excitement of the Queen's declaration of war against Russia. We had not advanced far enough in knowledge to ask them; and our fine troops went out destitute of sanitary care,—except such as was spontaneously bestowed by any qualified and benevolent person they might fall in with. One excellent thing was done in London, at the beginning of the year (1854), and before the troops embarked. The Head of the Medical Department of the army conversed with Lord Raglan on the peculiarities of climate, and of diseases, in the countries to which the troops were going; and, in consequence of that interview, the Director-General obtained leave from the Government to send out three commissioners to explore the localities in which the troops were likely to be encamped. Mr. A., Dr. B., and Dr. C., as we may call them, set out on their travels before the end of February. Mr. A. was to report of the country south and west of Adrianople, from Constantinople to the furthest probable western limit. Dr. B. followed the Danube from Vienna downwards, surveying its provinces, and coming out at Constantinople. He was to inquire into the diseases of the Principalities and of Turkey. Dr. C. was to examine the country usually traversed by forces bound for the Balkan and the North, from Constantinople, inquiring into climate, disease, and the features of the country, like his comrades. All were to consider the sites of camps, and to mark all particularly healthy or unhealthy spots. The instructions they carried must necessarily be meagre and vague, because the commission was new; but the scheme was a creditable one, and the three agents were evidently disposed to do their best. When it appeared that our force was to settle, in the first instance, at Gallipoli, a fourth commissioner, Dr. D., was sent there, with orders to examine and report of the town and neighbourhood, its water supply, and other particulars.

Commissioners' First Report.—While these gentlemen were on their travels, preparations went on busily at home; and while providing for sickness and wounds, the medical officer did not altogether forget health. He advised the sending out of a good supply of bell-tents and marquees, properly ventilated. He heard from Dr. B. from the Danube, that the Turkish troops at Widdin were wretchedly ill with fever and dysentery,—the place being marshy and unhealthy. The severity of the climate was great, and must be considered in the clothing of our troops. Unless they were dressed very differently from the ordinary mode, and well fed, and provided with abundance of bedding, they would die off like the Turks and Russians at that moment.

Immediate application was made at the War Office about the matter of clothing the troops. The red coat and the stiff leather stock would never do for summer wear; and flannel shirts and drawers, and worsted stockings were indispensable in cold and wet places. There should be a waterproof blouse, for ease of movement and coolness; and some headdress which would fend off the heat, and be light and well-fitting. If proposing were the same thing as achieving, here was something done in the sanitary department:— sites and water-supply ascertained; bedding, shelter, and clothing, all cared for, and plentiful food bespoken. The gap between proposing and achieving was not yet suspected.

Starting the Army.—Their Dress.—The day came for our soldiers to embark. Gallant enough they looked, as they marched to the railway stations, amidst the cheers and farewells of their countrymen, or passed on board ship, seeing a long line of waving handkerchiefs on the shore. We all remember those embarkations, and the satisfaction we felt in hearing of the good things provided with our money for our representative defenders. All the clothes were supposed to be new and right; every kit well supplied; and the transports loaded with whatever could be wanted in camp or on march. We were unaware that the cloth of the coats was harsh, so as to chafe, and stiffened with gum and size, so as to look substantial, but to be in reality a rag which let in the rain and the wind after a little wear; that the men's heads were hurt by their ill-fitting and heavy shakoes; that their boots were going into holes with a march of a few miles; and, above all, that breath and spirits were taken out of them by the oppression of the stock and the knapsack. The straps across the breast restricted the action of the lungs; and the leather round the throat brought on symptoms of apoplexy, in more or fewer soldiers, whenever an unusual march was required of them, or great exertion in hot weather. While it was our practice to confine our soldiers in barracks, without regular strenuous exercise, it was common for them to remark the decrease of their walking powers. A stout young peasant, who at home had thought nothing of carrying a load twenty miles, was astonished to find in a few months that he could scarcely keep up after a five miles' tramp in marching order. The tight coat, the choking stock, the straps on the chest, the pressure on the forehead, might account for it without supposing any great deterioration of health; though that was probable too.

It might have been known,—probably was known,—what mischief the stock had often done in hot countries; and the cases at home were enough for a warning:

yet our men went out with their throats so compressed. One of the medical officers could have told them, as he told the Sanitary Commission afterwards, what a sight it was, when, on a splendid day, the 60th Regiment was to enter King William's Town in Kaffraria, and many of the soldiers fell, within a space of a few yards, on the race-course. They had marched without their stocks, and were ordered to put them on, to enter the town: and this was the show they made! They were probably revived by instant relief being given; but it was otherwise in the Peninsular war. An old officer says it was heart-rending to see five men die in the space of little more than half a mile, mainly from the effects of the stock. Forty years later, however, we were shipping off other poor fellows, to drop under the summer sun of the East in the same way,— it being March and April when they left our shores.

Fate of the Exploring Commission.— A favourable voyage, and a hearty and admiring welcome at Malta, raised the spirits of the troops to a high pitch; and when they landed on Turkish territory, there was the amusement of fraternising with their French allies. They were disposed to make the best of everything in the gay new world they were introduced to; but bitter hardship awaited them from the very outset. Just when they were landing at Gallipoli, an answer was sent from London to the representation about suitable clothing and abundant bedding. The clothing could not be altered. The men could not have bedding; but it was hoped there was enough for the hospitals. The other recommendation of Dr. B., that there should be General Hospitals established in certain spots which he pointed out, was set aside by all parties. This was the result of one of the four preparatory missions. Nothing was ever heard of the reports of Mr. A., Dr. C., and Dr. D. The scheme of sanitary exploration proved altogether abortive. The explorers held no place, in fact, and were pushed aside for want of it. "The system" was not made for their admission; and the soldiers must take their chance of wet lodging, bad water, and no hospital to go to beyond their Regimental one, which could not be expanded to meet any extensive need.

The battalions landed at Gallipoli amidst fervid welcomes, but to encounter very cold nights, with the thermometer four degrees below freezing point. Where are the bell-tents? — the bedding we know was not allowed. "None could be sent." Perhaps it could and would have been sent, if it had been suspected how much more trouble and money it would cost to nurse, and lose, and bury the men who died for want of it.

The Peninsula of Gallipoli was chosen by the allies for their encampment, because it was considered a fit position for their depôts, their hospitals, and their stores. It was to be their base of operations: and there, of all places, our medical officers might reasonably expect to command everything necessary and comfortable for the sick. But there were no bell-tents: only a few marquees, and no other field equipments whatever. On those first freezing nights, the sick had but one single blanket to cover them; medical comforts could not be obtained, and the medical officer had to write to Malta for what he wanted on the very day of his arrival. Unable to obtain blankets for the sick in any other way, he seized them, and distributed them on his own responsibility.

Now, this was at the very outset of the war, when the Government believed, and the people of England took for granted, that everything was arranged for the welfare of the soldiery. The first step to destruction — the destruction of a truly noble army — was despising the aid of the four sanitary commissioners sent out beforehand.

A Sanitary Department needed. — What is the remedy? Is it not having a sanitary, as well as a medical, department for the army? Whether the two widely different functions should be conjoined in the same men is a question for discussion in another place. It is enough to say here, that some very important conditions must be fulfilled, if the offices are united in one profession. Whether so, or separate, the sanitary advisers must have some authority in the case — some rights as regards the military officials;

some means, in short, of doing their duty effectually. They cannot go out on commission to send in reports which are never heard of — to offer advice which is ignored — to point out requisites which are refused. Their element being once introduced into the governing council, to which is committed the *physique* of the army, the importance of preserving health, as well as restoring it, will be recognised, and the first great step will have been taken towards upholding the military strength of the empire, by modern science and art. By admitting a Minister of Health into the cabinet of the Director-General of the Army Medical Department, we may save (to take the lowest view) one third of the levies which we should require under a continuance of the old system. Other circumstances in the constitution of that cabinet will require notice hereafter.

Gallipoli. — The response from Malta to Gallipoli was not very exhilarating to the medical officers, whose patients were lying in the cold, comfortless and sinking. Three hundred sets of bedding, and some tents, were sent; but the medical comforts could not be allowed on the requisitions of the medical officers. It was a subject of complacency afterwards that there were so few sick at Gallipoli; and the number might have been expected to be larger under their actual misfortunes; but the lightness of the evil was certainly not owing to forethought grounded on knowledge. The knowledge did not, in fact, exist; and therefore such forethought as there was was desultory, unsupported, and almost entirely wasted. The medical service was declared by Ministers in Parliament to be "in the highest state of efficiency" at the time when the doctors were chafing and fretting over their inability to prevent the soldiers falling sick, in the first place, and to cure them in the next.

As has been seen, the suggestions of the Director-General about the clothing of the men, and the tents, were rejected at the outset. One other suggestion was accepted: — peat-charcoal, to the amount of 20 cwt., was sent to the medical officers in Turkey. Medicines were, of course, provided according to his judgment; but of consultation about the daily food, the dress, and the surrounding circumstances, there seems to have been none. The only intercourse between the military and medical authorities seems to have been about the clothing and tents, which were refused, and the peat-charcoal, which was granted.

Want of Concert. — The medical *chef* in London seems to have been equally silent towards the medical *chef* with the army. He seems to have had nothing to say about the diet of the soldiers, nor any other circumstance involving their health; nor did the *chef* in Turkey seem to have anything to ask of the *chef* in London, about diet or any other condition, till scurvy had become established in the camps. In like manner, the military *chef* did not resort for counsel to the medical *chef* about the nature and proportions of the food of the troops, or about their shelter or clothing; and he was not troubled with applications from the medical *chef* till the ravages of disease was almost past help. What happened in the higher official range happened below. There was no systematic consultation in the medical body; and the regimental commanders asked no counsel of their medical officers about the care of their men. There is nothing on record to show that any notion existed anywhere that the health of the army could be secured by the application of knowledge and care; and that it was of the utmost importance that it should be so secured. The idea was not, in fact, developed, nor at all admitted into our system of military preparation. Yet, where the Russians slew hundreds, epidemics slew their ten thousands.

Now that hygiene has been for some years recognised in civil life, and that every military system must include something analogous to its considerations, how do different methods work? In France, for instance. What is sanitary administration like there?

Sanitary Administration in France.—A Council of Health is attached to the Ministry of the Interior. This Council has no administrative power. When applied to by the Minister, it gives its opinion, which the Minister may act upon or not. Practically, he does almost invariably act upon it.

The Minister of War recurs in the same way to the advice of the medical council of the army; and the council is also required to volunteer its opinion whenever it may see occasion. It has no further power; and the Minister may act on its advice or not. As he often does not, the result is unsatisfactory, while in the civil case the method works well.

In England.—In England how is it? Our Home Office appoints Inspectors, who investigate, report, and offer recommendations. If these satisfy the Minister, he acts accordingly; if not, he returns the subject upon their hands for further consideration; and when satisfied, he proceeds upon them. The Interments' Act, and several others, show a beneficial result from this method;—and a very striking one, as the achievement of moving us out of our old ways, and troubling so many vested interests for so new a reason as the public health, appeared nearly hopeless beforehand.

The Board of Health, while it existed, did not get on so well. Its administrative principle was nearly the same; but it could not engage in conflict with whole communities, and override prejudices with so much advantage as a Secretary of State.

As to the War Office, we have seen what it is like in its communications with its Medical Department. The peat-charcoal was the one monument of its grace at our last entrance upon a great war. The most obvious consideration is that a department which will not attend to good advice will not long have a good adviser. An official who treats counsel on a special subject with disrespect, will not find respectable counsel at his command on special occasion. The four sanitary commissioners sent out before the last war, we have seen, were snubbed, and thereby silenced. The prodigious mortality which was the result might make any War Minister crave similar guidance next time; but it must be obtained by another Minister applying to another Inspector-General; unless the establishment of a sufficient sanitary organisation should meantime have rendered such a precaution a matter of course.

Difficulties.—It is true,—there are difficulties in the case. The War Office has many considerations to admit besides those which are all in all to the Medical Department. The British army is not sent abroad to promote its health, but to perform a war. Its health is an essential requisite; but it is not more: and the proceedings of the military authorities must be governed by a multitude of aims and reasons that the doctors know nothing about. To give the Director-General leave, therefore, to represent to the War Office all he thinks and wishes, would be not only to waste much time and trouble, but to cause him much needless mortification. In the late war, the Horse-Guards wrote a letter of thanks to the Medical Department which is very instructive in this connection. The advice was admirable, the letter says: but unfortunately it cannot be acted on. Such results must be frequent, if the Director-General were to speak whenever he had anything to say: and a few such failures would dishearten any man fit for such a charge as the *physique* of a national army.

Desiderata. — The true way would seem to be that suggested by the highest order of advisers,— that the Director-General should not volunteer his opinion. Scientific counsel, thrust upon an unscientific department, and not adopted, must soon become despicable. But, when the advice is asked, it should be on the understanding that, as a general rule, it will be acted upon. The Director-General, resorted to for an opinion which would be, in all probability, acted out, would be in a position of high responsibility, and his quality would probably correspond with his dignity; and the military authorities would be proportionably relieved of a responsibility for which they are not qualified. The thing would probably be done in this way. The Director-General would be put in possession of the case, as completely as the military authorities could furnish it, and be then asked, — "What ought we to do, under the circumstances, for the *physique* of the troops?" There can be no doubt that the authorities would be so glad of counsel on such occasions, as to be abundantly ready to adopt it.

It does not follow that the War Office need go

blundering on in the dark, in ignorance of hygienic considerations, except when expressly asking for advice. To give information is one thing, and to offer an opinion is another. The War Office ought to be glad of any possible amount of information from all reliable sources; and particularly of a special kind of information from scientific authority. The Director-General should therefore have freedom and inducement to communicate hygienic information to the Minister of War, — the times and seasons of communication being arranged for the convenience of the office.

These are the conclusions arrived at by those who best know how to utilise the experience of the late war; and they will probably be adopted and made practical. One recommendation of the method to the national feeling and judgment would be that, in case of failure, there could be no doubt where the responsibility rested. If the War Office had asked and obtained, and acted upon scientific advice, the advising department would be called to account. At present, the Director-General says what he thinks; the War Office listens or ignores; and when an enormous mortality ensues, there is no discovering where the responsibility lies. It is shifted about till all that can be done is to lay the blame on "the system," — or the absence of system, — and let the officials escape. This may be the fairest conclusion on a single occasion: but the method will not bear repetition.

The relations between the military and medical authorities at the seat of war should be the same as those at home. The General in command and the medical *chef* should be on the same footing:—the physician affording information to the General at fitting times, and his counsel when asked. The position authorises a somewhat larger liberty to the physician, inasmuch as his knowledge of local sanitary circumstances must be greater than that of the military *chef*, whose strategy must ordinarily be largely affected by them, and may occasionally be entirely dependent on them for success or failure. Again, in smaller divisions of the force, down to the lowest, it should be understood that the same relations exist. Thus may the hygienic ignorance of military officers be counteracted in its most fatal effects; while the responsibility of the advisers is reduced in proportion to their fitness for their function. If, further, it should be made obligatory on the sanitary officials to communicate among themselves, so as to throw their knowledge into a common stock, and on the military officials to report to the War Department their reasons for rejecting sanitary or medical advice, we shall probably have secured the protection of the *physique* of the army, as far as the relations of the military and medical authorities in strategical matters can effect it.

First Camp.—When our troops landed at Gallipoli, however, all affairs of this kind were at sixes and sevens. The French were there before us. They had very naturally settled themselves to their liking: and they had a custom of shifting their encampments nearly every fortnight, which answered two good purposes at least. It set the soldiers down on new ground, clean (comparatively), fresh, and requiring salutary labour, and it obviated panic in case of any removal being required by sanitary alarms. If the enemy spread any false rumour about the site of the camp — that it had been a plague-field, or a cemetery, or what not — the French could be moved a few days sooner, or at short notice, without anything like the panic to which the British were liable, who were not accustomed to break up their camp without some solemn reason. The lines at Gallipoli were to extend seven miles from the old town; and thence it was supposed were the allies to operate during the war. It was to be their base of operations; and there they were to threaten the right flank of the Russians, if the Russians were to threaten Constantinople. So there the British and French soldiers fraternised at once with a warmth which troubled their doctors. The Highlander and the Zouave drank to their eternal friendship till they found themselves in a sorrowful pickle,— the Zouave in kilt and bonnet, and the Highlander in a wonderful red and blue disguise, through which his tartan hose made a ludicrous disclosure of his identity. The mixed uniforms were a joke; but the drunkenness and its consequences were no joke. The amount of the vice, the vile quality of the spirit obtained by the soldiers, and the sickness which ensued, caused the first anxiety about the war to those in command and at home. When twenty culprits, sick and stupified from drink, were brought up for judgment from one regiment in one morning, the medical men might well be anxious and dismayed. Then, too, they became acquainted with the conditions of Turkish buildings, from barracks to hovels. The vermin, the decaying wood, the accumulated filth, the evil scents within, and the bones and offal without, promised everything bad. The dry dusty ravines in the neighbourhood, with the wretched villages of the peninsula scattered among them, were the very picture of desolation, choked with rubbish, and resounding with the howlings of curs, assembled to devour any dead animal which had come to lay its bones there. The magnates of the forces reviewed the troops, looked at the tents, tasted the rations, and approved everything; but it must have been a relief to the medical officers when the long field-works at Gallipoli were abandoned, and the troops were removed — the British to Scutari, and the French to the neighbourhood of Constantinople.

Varna.— By the end of May, the allied forces were landing at Varna for their next long sojourn. Few had any idea of what ravage could happen there without a shot being fired. A narrow beach lay between the sea and the town wall; and on this beach lay enormous quantities of ammunition. The town itself was soon brightened and ventilated by the French, who threw down old walls, opened new streets, set up a post-office and other establishments, and put out of sight an inconceivable amount of dirt, so that the natural impression was of the place being wholesome. We at home heard much of the beauty and value of the neighbouring hills as sites for encampment. Within the enclosed space lying between the northern and southern ranges there was a considerable variety of scenery, a pretty lake westwards of the town, rising grounds, soon overspread with the tents of the allies, and the greenest of plains affording waterfowl for the officers' sport, and so on. These plains being swamps, no doubt there were plenty of aquatic birds. The rising grounds were not out of the reach of marsh exhalations; and the junction at the westwards of the surrounding hills precluded any sufficient ventilation. A high barrier, overgrown at its base with brushwood, shut in an area of undrained land, sodden by the overflow of lake and streams, meeting the salt waves of the Euxine. When the troops had been there two months, we at home, after admiring the sketches and descriptions we received from young poets and sportsmen, began to wonder whether any older heads had dissented from the general approbation of the site. The Quartermaster-General naturally looks first for wood and water, and so far this was a favourable spot. But what said the doctors? There was not much encouragement to them to say anything. One of them had already ventured to give the information that the sickness in his division was clearly traceable to the parade being at noon, instead of in the cool hours: and the answer he got was that when his advice was desired he would be asked for it. If, on arriving at Varna, he had pointed out the stagnant waters and the stagnant air, he would probably have encountered a repetition of the rebuff. Military reasons override all others in such a case, no doubt. The thing to be desired is that sanitary considerations should enter among military reasons henceforth, and the supply of pure air be as much made a point of as an abundance of wood and water.

Of many suggestions made directly to Lord Raglan, several were attended to. Noonday-drill, bad spirits and sour wine, sameness of rations, exposure of sentries to the sun, sale of bad meat, causes of foul smells, were all brought before him; and with good effect, for the most part. Porter was promised; but it never arrived. It was provided by Government; but it was kept back "for want of transport," though it could have been easily sent. The men were ordered beef and mutton alternately; their heads were to have white coverings as the summer heats came on; sentries were to be under cover, and fatigue parties more frequently relieved. But a week or two showed how much more was wanted to save the force from destruction.

So early as the 6th of June, the Deputy-Inspector-General of Hospitals asked for mattrasses and various medical comforts for two hundred men who had "literally nothing." Four days after, he represented the destitute state of the sick,—such an absolute want of medicines, equipments and comforts as would make their condition dreadful, if the army should have to move. The letter was pronounced disagreeable; and the writer was recommended to keep his suggestions to himself till they were asked for. It was not explained how the commanders were to know that the hospitals were properly supplied, if not from the Inspector of Hospitals. It was not till the 18th that the anxious Inspector was informed that the supplies would be sent.

The Cholera.—Meantime the cholera had appeared. The first case occurred on the 18th of June. The soldiers were drinking sour country wine, eating stone fruit and cucumbers, and sugar adulterated with sand (one of the most mischievous of the abuses mentioned), uncovering their heads in the sun, bathing upon an insufficient breakfast, and longing for good vegetables, which were not to be had. Now came on the first gloom,—the skirts of that black cloud which was about to overshadow our fortunes in our eastern war.

As diarrhœa spread among the soldiers, they were

desired to apply at once to the doctors. Some did, some did not. On the 3rd of July, morning drill began;—5 A.M., instead of noon. Orderlies were supplied to the hospital; but certain defects in the place were never remedied. On the 9th, small-pox was reported from one of the villages, and the men were forbidden to go there. On the same day, three cases of cholera were reported from the Devna Camp. From that date, the scene is truly dreary to read of, from one end of our encampments to the other. It was on a Sunday that the first Devna case occurred; and rumours spread of many having died of it. It at once became a question whether to move the camp; —or rather, when to move it. The French could have shifted their ground, briskly and gaily, at once, as they were used to the movement; but it would be death to the British to be panic-stricken by hasty and unusual measures. It was evident in an hour or two, however, that the panic of remaining would be the worst of the two. The soldiers exclaimed that the site was condemned by the Inspector; horrible reports got abroad of what the place had been; and the men declared that not one of them would survive if they remained. So they were taken to Monastir, whence was sent a singular series of letters from the medical officer in charge to the responsible medical officer at Varna.

Monastir was called the Montpelier of Bulgaria; but the disease spread fearfully. The appeals for medicine and comforts became urgent before the end of the month. Two and three letters a day asked for arrow-root, brandy, opium, naphtha, hydrocyanic acid: the wine was all but gone; brandy had been bought because it was impossible to wait. Again, the opium and brandy, &c., must be sent immediately: the need is most urgent; a horse araba, (horse and cart) could bring them. After four and five days, nothing has arrived, — cholera is raging, — surely the orderly dragoon could bring the medicines. Next day, an orderly is sent to Varna with a longer list of needs, and a note of the preceding unanswered letters. Camphor, laudanum, mustard, ammonia, turpentine, and other medicines; and arrow-root, wine, brandy, sago, are all exhausted, and nothing has arrived. Next day, the same thing again; — an early and large supply is requested, the same day or next morning early, by some mule waggons. And what was the answer? Five thousand cholera belts (the first article asked for), and a request for more accurate reports of the health of the division! A few articles followed the cholera belts the next day, when the petitioning letters began to arrive; but the supplies were exhausted before more were received; and meantime the cholera had spread to the artillery. While toiling among his hourly multiplying patients, without medicines or proper food, the unhappy physician received from Varna complaints of the "lavish use of arrcw-root and other articles;"— as if the object were not to restore the sick at any cost of arrow-root! "Unexpected demand"—"store exhausted"—"quest in Constantinople"—"requisition to England"—for articles of prime necessity, on which the very life of the army depended! The remonstrance on "lavish use" was accompanied by a lecture to the toil-worn physician, who had a whole plague upon his hands, on precision as to dates and facts in replying to inquiries;—a lecture for future use, apparently, as it was not applicable at the moment.

The military authorities found the same kind of need and anxiety on every hand; and some of them spoke out plainly as to unnecessary delays in affording supplies. Yet, there is a letter on record, dated the 13th of August, by which the harassed physician is informed that his "requisition for medicine has been ready for two or three days; but, as it is not a load for an araba," there were no means of despatching it. While men were dying by hundreds for want of a spoonful of medicine each, the medicine could not be sent, because it was not a load for a cart! If a bat-horse was sent in with panniers, that would be a good plan, it was suggested. A dozen lost soldiers are somewhat more costly than the hire of a cart. This letter was crossed by one from the physician, informing the authorities that he had been obliged to divide the remnant of his stores with the Cavalry Brigade, which was "completely run out of everything." After more correspondence about a pack-horse for the medicines ("which hardly require an araba"), and a hint to use ground rice for arrow-root, the araba was at last (on the 17th of August) sent, with medicines, wine, brandy and ground rice; and it is acknowledged as bringing "some few medicines and comforts." The requisition for these had been acknowledged from Varna on the 7th; and it was the 18th before they arrived! The Commissariat would have furnished a mule-cart at any moment, if requested. It has been remarked, that between the two objections, that loads are too heavy and too light for a cart, the soldiers have many a time suffered grievously.

After all, there was no port-wine in the cart; the purveyor had omitted it. Porter was requested; and the wine and porter were at length provided. Thus went on the epidemic and the doctors in Bulgaria.

At Varna, fatigue parties were busy burying the dead. The troops, English and French, grew listless and despondent — did not know nor care where they should go next — would certainly die if they remained here — heard things were just as bad on board the fleet — had not expected to be sacrificed wholesale before even seeing the enemy. Then occurred the great fire, which consumed a vast amount of stores. Our sailors put it out, after ten hours of extraordinary exertion. Then, again, the dwindling regiments sat watching the spread of the grave-yards, and the passage of funerals all day long.

The best of our soldiers had sunk to being obliged to divide a march of ten miles between two days. The strongest staggered under their knapsacks. Arrangements were knocked up by the disappearance of whole bodies of functionaries; as the drivers of the ambulance corps. When we, at home, canvassed that autumn the policy of the Crimean expedition, we little dreamed that such a consideration was involved as the very existence of our army in the East. But so it was.

The migration to the Crimea saved our force; and was only just in time. The men were so weak that they could scarcely carry their own weight. Hence the loss of their kits, and of many things which they would not, on landing, have believed they could throw away. We are told that in another month not a man would have remained alive.

Moral. — After all that has been said, and can be said, about the want of organisation in the medical service, and of sense and foresight in providing for visitations of sickness, it remains true that the deficiency of a sanitary department was a graver misfortune still. It happened through ignorance. We know better now; and it is inconceivable that a British army should ever again sit down in a malarious valley, for want of a Department whose business it should be to secure the army from epidemics, as the Commissariat secures it from starvation.

CHAP. IV.

MEETING THE ENEMY.

THE best medicine that the sinking forces could have was the news that they were going to meet the enemy. It is well that they had it; for no medicines nor medical comforts were sent out from England from May 27th to September 20th. The probable need had been miscalculated; and there was no end to the wonder where all the good things could have gone to, though the sick were in September 11,000 instead of the 2000 which had been reckoned on. What could have become of the opium and the brandy and the arrow-root, was a sore puzzle to those who had been completely deceived as to the important considerations of numbers and quantities. We shall see hereafter how defective the statistics of disease, and indeed all statistics, were, and how much depends on a department which could not then be said to exist. At present, however, we have not done with the subject of the need of concert and communication between the military and the medical officers, and between the medical officers themselves.

Want of Concert.—It seems to have been during

the abode in Bulgaria that the medical officers began to apprehend that they must take charge of the health, as well as the sickness of the troops. There was not yet any regular inquisition as to the quality of food, or interference as to lodging and its site. This was nobody's business; and therefore it was not done. But there was some activity about the treatment of nuisances, and more frequent application to Lord Raglan, as time went on. It was too late now to encamp the men on the table-lands north and south of the swamp they were in, or to undo the mischief of unwholesome food; but there are signs of an awakening to the importance of considerations which there was no department to provide for. Want of concert between the different departments destroyed their ability to make up for a deficient one; but the sense of the deficiency was beginning to grow, and first on the medical side, judging from the fact that the doctors were left without notice when the army was going to move. Even the *chef* of the department "received no intelligence at all that the army was about to embark from Varna." There had been rumours in the camps for some time; but the first notice to be making ready was two thousand sick being thrown upon the department, to be carried somewhere in a trice. No doubt it was a secret when and where the army was to go; but heads of departments must be taken into the secret in such cases, if they are to do their duty. At the last moment some of the ships had two doctors, and some three, and some none at all. Some had medicines, and some had none. So much for the 2000 existing sick,—to say nothing of the prospective wounded, now that the enemy was to be met.

The medical *chef* at once made application for the transport of 400 tons of stores, which were absolutely necessary. He had only four days to make the entire preparations for the Crimean campaign. The stores were brought by country carts through the narrow streets of Varna; and when they were on the beach, there were no means of getting them on board. Lord Raglan had happened to mention in conversation the name of the vessel which was to take them; and this saved them from being left behind. Boats were obtained: and when half the stores were on board, the physician was duly informed of the name of the ship. There was not the same luck throughout. One surgeon tells us how his regiment was obliged to leave behind at Varna the new regimental medicine-chest, provided for service of this very kind, and was allowed to carry only two panniers full of medicines and surgical instruments, with a marquee and two hospital canteens. No ambulance, no means of conveyance were allowed but ten stretchers, to be conveyed by the band,—already well loaded. Lord Raglan was appealed to, by the medical *chef*, on the matter of ambulance provision; and he caused twelve waggons to be shipped complete for use. He sailed before the transport, however, and "some one" objected to the arrangement, and ordered the waggons to be put on shore again. Ten were landed, the mules of all were drowned, and the harness was lost: so that two waggons, without draught and harness, represented the ambulance of Lord Raglan's force when it went out to meet the enemy. This was at a time when the soldiers could not accomplish a march of ten miles without their knapsacks; and when, at the same time, they were expected to encounter the enemy at their landing-place. With the unwounded too weak to march, with their own comforts on their shoulders, and the wounded unprovided with means of conveyance, what was to become of the 20,000 British soldiers starting for the Crimea?

Such was the prospect, through want of organisation and concert. It had never been settled who had a right to speak, and whose duty it was to inquire and to reply.

The Voyage. — The voyage was got over more easily than could have been expected, — more prosperously than by our allies. Our soldiers were less crowded in the transports than the French; and though we had many sick, there was no such mortality as on board the French ships. In both cases there was every advantage that exhilaration could give; for the troops were in the highest spirits at the prospect of action, after four or five months of conflict with mere disease.

Old Fort.—Not an enemy was in sight, however, till that cool Russian officer whom we all remember, as a capital specimen of a first foe, with his Cossack attendants, appeared approaching the sea-shore, dismounted, and sat down to make notes, or a sketch, of what was doing. We all remember him, and the snatch made by his Cossacks at Sir George Brown and his staff; and not less clearly do we recall the scenery,—so dreary in description, and so exhilarating to the men who had escaped from the Bulgarian plague-trap. Was it not that night that the Duke of Cambridge crept under a waggon for shelter from the drenching rain? The French soldiers had *tentes d'abri,*—coverings which two soldiers could easily carry in halves, and put together for their shelter from rain and noon sunshine,—but our poor fellows lay in the rain. At a later time they were abundantly willing to add a pound and a half to the weight of their load for the benefit of such shelter; but the method was then unknown to us.

At Old Fort, then, on the 14th of September, lay our twenty thousand men, with the sea outside, and the salt lakes inside of the sandy spit on which they had, in such perfect order and silence, landed themselves, their thirty-six guns, and their multitude of horses.

The Sick.— How were the sick to be conveyed? It was said that the ambulance waggons were too heavy, if they could have been brought; but they were broken to pieces long ago. The corps of drivers had dropped and died, or disappeared. What could be done with the sick? It was very late to be thinking of this.

Before the force left Old Fort, the hospital marquee and canteens before spoken of were re-embarked by order; and only four water mules remained for the whole battalion reported of by its medical officer. Only one circular tent was allowed for a whole regiment. Some country people ran away at the sight of a picket of ours, leaving their carts behind them; these rude carts were of great value at such a moment, and they formed the nucleus of a native transport corps. The want of concert, which made such a windfall so precious, seems scarcely intelligible; but it is on record that the sick and weakly seemed to be thrown over to the mercies of chance, — unremembered by the military authorities, and not much the better for the indignation and pity which raged in the hearts of their willing but helpless doctors. The lagging of the sick and feeble, — their dropping behind, — their sinking on the road, and the trail of corpses where the army had marched, were features of the first going out to meet the enemy. It would be hard to bear the thought now, but for the assurance we for the first time possess that such a desultory way of going to war can never be witnessed again.

First March.—It was on the 19th that the force advanced in search of a more substantial enemy than

Tartar peasants and Cossack scouts. The men were already pretty well tired of their first resting-place in the Crimea. When the sun shone, they were scrambling about the water-tub for the draught they were fainting for want of; and when it rained, they soon had more than enough of it. They lay in puddles and mud all night; and during the day were running into the sea at every opportunity, for the chance of drying their clothes on the beach. On the night of the 18th every man knew that he was to move on the morrow; and all seemed to rise with a will when the *reveille* sounded at 3 A.M. The ships' boats were presently in line along the shore; the soldiers piled on the beach everything that could possibly be spared; and the sailors tossed into the boats the knapsacks, and many other necessaries, which it was fatal to a sick soldiery to part with, but which the men were too weak to carry, and there were no means of carrying otherwise. Amidst the bustle of sending most of the baggage to the ships, and struggling to forward the rest, and the necessary food, by a beggarly array of carts, all would have looked like hopeless confusion, but for the regiments which were parading, in preparation for the march, as steadily as if they had been in Hyde Park. It was nine o'clock before all was ready for the start.

There was no road. Tracks over the dry and dreary steppe were the only signs of habitation for many a mile. The Turkish soldiers were gone forwards next the beach, and the French next to the Turks. The British were in a more dangerous position than either, — further inland, and sure to be the first assailed by an enemy on the watch. Not a tree or a shrub was to be seen, except at some remote village inland; and there was no shelter from the burning sun, or relief from the monotony of the march. Low ridges crossed the track, one after another; and as each was passed, there was an eager out-look for water, always in vain. It was no wonder that the sick fainted, and the weak fell out. The march was not a long one; but there was an increase of cholera and dysentery at the end of it. Lord Raglan called that march "most wearisome;" and said that the men were "pursued by cholera to the very battle-field." Yet they were full of ardour at the first halt, before noon, and cheered and sprang forward when their general rode along the front, though they were parched with thirst. They chased, during their halts, the hares they started, — the only living things left by the enemy along their route; and at three o'clock they lighted upon something more acceptable, — the muddy little river Bulganac, which flowed seawards across their track. The soldiers sprang at the water as at a prey.

That night, again, was, by Lord Raglan's account, a very trying one. It was, according to that statement, a choice between bringing soldiers or baggage animals; and the soldiers were considered the most necessary. "My anxiety to bring into the country," wrote Lord Raglan, in his despatch of September 23rd, " every cavalry and infantry soldier who was available, prevented me from embarking their baggage animals; and these officers have with them at this moment nothing but what they can carry; and they, equally with the men, are without tents or covering of any kind. I have not heard a single murmur." " Since the men landed," he says, " they have been exposed to the extremes of wet, cold, and heat; and the daily toil to provide themselves with water has been excessive." Yet, if the men sank to the ground, there they must lie, as the necessary aids were out of reach, though within view. They were on board those ships, five miles to the west, which were holding a parallel course to the march, — the lines of smoke at sea and of glittering arms on land appearing to telegraph each other. A mile beyond the Bulganac, the force halted for the night; and just in front the first blood was shed, — four of the cavalry being wounded in a skirmish on the ground which was to become illustrious next day, as the scene of the battle of the Alma.

First Bivouac on March.— The tired men collected furze and weeds for their fires, which were soon fed with casks as they were emptied of salt meat and rum. All night the straggling carts were coming up, and such of the men as were able to overtake their comrades. The night was damp and cold; and after the scorching day, the men lay exposed, with only their coats and an occasional blanket for a covering. For three weeks more the troops must sleep in this way. The tents were not issued till the middle of October.

It is difficult to understand why a certain amount of transport has not always been, as a matter of course, allotted to regiments on march, as an article of the first necessity. On the beach at Varna there were stores lying about with the hospital mark on them, which nobody knew what to do with for want of means to remove them. In the Crimea the surgeons caught any country cart they could lay hands on, to carry the panniers of medicines and instruments. They were happy if they proceeded unchallenged. If the vehicle was wanted for the baggage of the staff* the panniers must turn out, and be left behind, unless good luck should send another cart that way. Where there is due concert between the military and the medical authorities, each regiment should be as secure of the carriage of its hospital stores, and of vehicles for the sick and weakly, as of its meat and drink. The battle of the Alma was won because British soldiers can resist the discouragements of sickness and privation as long as resistance is possible; but if the day at the Alma had been lost, it would have been because there had

* Evidence, p. 81, Q. 2626.

been no well-arranged guardianship of the men's health. It was owing to want of concert that the men were staggering on their feet, and dizzy in their march, till the spirit of the hour acted on them like a cordial; and if that spirit had been a whit less willing, the flesh was so weak that anybody might have conquered our troops; and the disgrace would not have rested with the soldiers, — as the glory happily does. "Pursued by cholera to the battle-field," should always be quoted (from Lord Raglan's despatch) when the action is described, and the conduct of our novice soldiers commemorated. "In the ardour of attack, they forgot all they had endured." That was it; and it is the strongest possible appeal to us to take care that sickness on a march is never again left out of view in the arrangements.

The Battle.—The full horror of it was after the battle. Was there ever a more impressive contrast than the field presented within three days!

No bugles or drums roused the British force for the battle,—the first battle of most of the men there. Their Commander's memory was thronged with the imagery of Peninsular conflicts, and of the last great battle of the world, which had brought forty years of peace: but, except a few veterans of Lord Raglan's standing, there was not a man there who had witnessed a fight in Europe. To those who had been in the Sikh war, the scene was almost as new. All were alike aware that this day would be marked in history as that of the first battle after Waterloo; and high beat thousands of hearts at the thought. They were roused and formed by the light of the watch-fires; and the hum of many thousand voices might have been heard a long way through the fog, though not so far as the Russians. When a light breeze carried off the fog, the ships were seen between the hills already in motion along the shore; the generals were riding along the lines, and meeting and parting, as they made and communicated their last arrangements; and then, when the sun revealed the whole scheme, the bugles and drums burst into clangour, and made many pulses beat as they never beat before. When the mist cleared from the opposite heights, the stillness appeared so complete that the Russians were supposed to have retired from their position. It was far otherwise, however. The position was a strong one; and the Russians had such confidence in it that the thought of defeat seems not to have occurred to them. Spectators from Sebastopol were on the ridge,—come out to see the discomfiture of the allies as they would have gone to a tournament, a few centuries earlier. As the light penetrated under the fog, the allies saw two dark masses forming gradually behind the principal battery, and lines of cavalry and infantry extending on the heights above. Fleet horsemen were scudding about in the plain below; and statue-like sentinels occupied the best posts of observation.

Next after the ships of the allies, the French advanced; and at ten o'clock the impatient British were allowed to start. Their scarlet lines and squares moving down the slopes, with the artillery between the divisions, and the rifles and light cavalry protecting the front and left flank, and forests of bayonets flashing in the sun, from the eastern moorland to the sea, made up a gallant sight, to be the last on earth that many present looked upon. Then followed the halting in line as the divisions came up with the French, and with each other; and the retreat of the Cossack videttes across the stream, after firing the village of Burliuk; and the feat remained which the Russians considered impossible,—that of crossing the Alma below the slopes occupied by the enemy, and driving them up the steps and over the ridge. To thousands of men in each of the assembled forces it must have appeared impracticable, considering the high banks of the stream, and the rocks and ravines, penetrated only by rough tracks, scarcely passable for any kind of vehicle in the most fair weather circumstances, and now occupied or commanded by a countless soldiery, or an array of artillery of most formidable quality, and precisely acquainted with the range of all the points below and around. The prospect was as desperate as the Russians concluded it to be. Yet, at an hour past noon, the Zouaves were bursting from the brushwood across the river, near its mouth, and spreading and climbing over the heights on the seaward flank of the Russians;—"swarming like ants" over the steep face of the cliff, and reaching the heights, to the consternation of the Cossacks below, who found themselves between two foes, and, with their artillery and infantry, made way for the main body of the French to follow to the support of their own skirmishers. The wonderful work of carrying up the artillery was accomplished. On the upland, the conflict was fierce; and especially about a tumulus which the Russians contested staunchly, but on which the French flag was reared by a Zouave sergeant who fought with a monkey on his shoulder. He was shot down in the act, bequeathed his pet to the care of his comrades, and died. The monkey is said to have gone gallantly through the war; but we cannot but wish it had been the victim.

The Russians directed such a force against the victorious French, that the arrangements of the commanders were somewhat changed, and the British were ordered forwards sooner than the moment appointed. On they went against desperate odds,—against masses on the slopes, batteries at every point of advantage, and marksmen hidden in vineyards, brushwood, and ravines. Lord Raglan and his staff plunged into the ford, and, in the midst of a perfect hail of shot and shell, the whole force floundered through, at one point or another, in deeper or shallower water, and below more or less formidable banks. Up they rushed and scrambled to the cannon's mouth in the redoubt which cost so many lives. Barely able to hold their ground amidst their heaps of dead, on this the central spot of the action of the day, the British saw a compact mass of Russian infantry marching down upon them. If they ever arrived, the day was lost. Then was heard Lord Raglan's question whether a couple of guns could be brought to bear on that moving square: then was the effort made, and the guns came up: then was the first shot seen to miss; but next was the fortune of the day seen to turn,—the shot seen to make lanes through the mass,—the mass seen to waver and break, and disperse in flight over the ridge. After that there was no more doubt about driving the Russians over the crest. The splendid charge up the steep went on irresistibly; and when the allies stood on the ridge, the French turned the guns they found there on the flying foe. The battle of the Alma was over. Of our infantry two divisions were never engaged. The other 14,000 encountered 20,000 Russians; and the proportion of numbers between the French and Russians was about the same.

The British now knew what a great battle was. Their losses were larger than the French, through the fierceness of the conflict before the redoubt: they were much smaller than the Russian loss; but grave enough to prevent any man present ever forgetting that day. We lost 362 killed, and 1640 were wounded. There they lay on the red sodden soil, while many a comrade sent word home of how nobly they had helped to win so great a victory!

After the Battle. — What a contrast, as I said, did that valley present within the few hours between the reaching and the leaving it! First, was there any other place so glorious, with its meeting armies, its tread of numbers, and its clash of war-music, and uproar of cheers! Soon after, was there any other place so desolate and forlorn? The army was gone, "over the hills and far away;" and the fleet was gone. The heroes were not all gone. One or two whose names should be immortal were there,—Surgeon Thomson and his assistant, who saw the troops disappear over the ridge, leaving them to do what two men could for seven hundred wounded Russians, with no defence against a swoop of the enemy, if the Cossack scouts on the hills should see them at their work. During two days from the disappearance of the Russians, our soldiers, aided by the sailors, had been busy removing the wounded to the ships, each in a hammock, slung to an oar, and carried by four men; or in burying the dead. But long before all this was done, they must march again; and Dr. Thomson and his assistant were left with the seven hundred Russians, who must have perished but for their devotedness. If ever devotedness was put to the proof it must have been in that blood-sodden valley, amidst the ruins of burnt dwellings, where all was silence, except for the groans of the wounded, and where the sufferers and their benefactors could not communicate, from having no common language. Dr. Thomson died; and no doubt all England mourned him.

To Sebastopol. — Meanwhile, the forces were moving on. Over the Katscha, over the Belbek they marched, — still dropping cholera patients as they went. More and more sufferers from dysentery were sent to the rear. As the country became less wild, the soldiers found more amusement and somewhat better fare; but still disease haunted them. They found grapes, melons, and other fruits, and many vegetables, in the gardens of country-houses, and ate largely of them. When exhausted by marches through tangled woods, or the pathless steppe, they drank whatever came in their way. They made light of warnings, — both of advice and of premonitory symptoms; and the next thing was being sent to the rear and becoming helpless. How Lieutenant Maxse succeeded in breaking his way through the wood in the course of a night march, after the fatigues of the day, and sent round the Admiral to meet the General at Balaclava, where they arrived at the same moment, we do not forget: nor how a large division of the Russian force was scattered by a handful of our troops coming out of the wood; but, notwithstanding the brave acts that were done, and the fortunate incidents which occurred, our soldiers were sorely sick and suffering when the Allies sat down before Sebastopol.

Hospitals. — What was it that was done with the sick and wounded? They were sent to the rear; but what was in the rear? What became of them, in short? If they had had all the transport that could have been desired, — vehicles, with good mules, cork mattrasses and bedding, and carts to pick up fainting stragglers, — what next? The answer is, that they were taken, like the wounded at Alma, to a Field-hospital. What is a Field hospital? It is any sheltered place in which the sufferers can be collected for convenience of treatment and protection. If nothing better offers, tents are the natural resource; and a provision of tents for the wounded and sick seems to be one of the first ideas that would occur to authorities planning a battle or a march. A Field-hospital signifies, — means on the spot for taking care of the sick and wounded.

A Regimental hospital is the place in which the sick and wounded of a regiment are collected, to be treated by the medical men of the regiment. Our military commanders have always preferred Regimental hospitals to any other method of dealing with the sick; and it is probably the best way under ordinary circumstances at home, and favourable conditions abroad. But it is obvious at a glance that, under an attack of a virulent epidemic, or after a sanguinary battle, the Regimental hospital must break down from insufficiency. There can be no chance for the sufferers when half the regiment is down in cholera, or a third or two-thirds wounded. The organisation is not adequate to the strain upon it in such critical circumstances; and critical circumstances are precisely what it is the business of the military art to provide against. There must clearly be some resource for the Regimental hospitals to fall back upon.

General Hospitals. — General Hospitals are that resource. Military commanders admit it with great reluctance; and, indeed, it seems like a melancholy satire to give the name of a resource to an establishment which has been invested with so bad a name, and such painful associations, as our General Hospitals have been through many wars. Sufferers have entered them only to die. Such was the popular belief in the army in the Peninsular and other wars; and such is the avowal of grieved and perplexed commanders in moments of confidence. After many attempts to do without them, always ending in a final, hopeless recourse to them, the necessity of General Hospitals has been admitted by all authorities, the preference still attaching to the Regimental hospitals.

Is such a dilemma as this necessary? Is there no escape from such a perplexity? Knowledge and painstaking have solved the difficulty; and hence issues one of the broadest lights by which our future military prospect is cheered.

The idea of what a Military General Hospital ought to be is new; — new in clearness, and new in practice; but it is so ascertained as never again to be lost. Till recently, a Military General Hospital was simply a cluster of Regimental hospitals. Sick and wounded were stowed into one place, or group of places, and treated according to the accidental means of the moment, without the benefit of anything that could be called organisation and unity of control. It is now made plain, by study and experience, that one of the first considerations in entering upon a campaign, is to provide, at the base of operations, a General Hospital of sufficient capacity to meet any calls that can be anticipated; and so commanded and organised in each department, as to allow the utmost chance of recovery to all who enter it. By practice during peace, and timely arrangements in prospect of war, the institution should be open for use on the first gun-fire, or the first attack of sickness. There every patient who arrives should be at once received into a system which, by steady laws, supplies him with good air, nursing, diet, and medical care, so that the controllable influences may all tend to his recovery. With such an institution in the background, in which to deposit the long cases, and the most serious (if a clearance has to be made of the lighter), the Regimental hospitals may prosper to the utmost in undertaking the briefer and less grave maladies and wounds. In such modes of warfare as involve long sieges or many battles, there may be a necessity for several General Hospitals, as we found in the late war. Wherever they are, and whatever their size, their distinctive feature is the organisation by which the great functions of tending the sick are performed, as by natural laws, in contrast to the desultory methods of Regimental hospitals, where an assemblage of sick and wounded soldiers are individually provided for, under their own medical officers and by their own immediate comrades.

We shall see, hereafter, what the great hospital at the base of operations was like at the outset of the late war. At present we have to consider the case of the sick and wounded in the Crimea after the battle of the Alma, in order to learn what precautions should be taken about the disposal of such sufferers.

Sick Transport.—It seems to have been about the 3rd of August that the transport of the sick and wounded first seriously occupied the attention of the chief medical authorities on the spot, — that is, at Varna. We have seen what became of the waggons that were shipped under the orders of the Commander-in-Chief. The ambulance service broke down immediately. The vehicles themselves broke down; and the incompetent drivers and attendants vanished.

Two or three of the vehicles reappeared before Sebastopol at a subsequent time, when the mud had been got rid of. During the reign of the mud, the sufferers were removed by dragoon horses, mules and pack-horses, and litters and mules lent by our allies, to a General Hospital established at Balaclava, — shortening the travels of the sick. The new Land Transport department undertook the work afterwards; but, at the first landing in the Crimea, the sick seem to have been thrown upon the mercies of chance, while attended by anxious and devoted surgeons, who were themselves rather the victims than the perpetrators of the mistake. According to the rules of the army, the medical department is dependent on other departments for ambulance and transport of the sick and wounded: and there is plenty of evidence of the earnestness with which the surgeons petitioned for it.

When the army was taken to a peninsula, which was all but an island, to invade it, and besiege its stronghold, one of the leading considerations would naturally be how to send away the helpless. We had a fleet there. The Quarter-master-general and naval commanders, one would think, would consult with the chief medical officer present about where and how to embark the seriously sick and wounded, how to provide for them on board the ships, and where to take them to. Those who could not bear a long voyage, and those who might become fit for action again, would be taken to the General Hospital at the base of operations, while the permanently disabled should be sent home by the first opportunity. This is seen now to be the reasonable method; but nothing of the sort was done. There was no organisation. When wants were perceived, they were urged, and attempts were made to supply them; but the sufferers were dead before the supplies came. Between Old Fort and the Alma, there were the ships moving along the coast, with the few marquees, tents, and stores of the expedition on board: and on land were the 20,000 British, marching in the heat, and dropping with cholera by the way, and no shelter or comforts for them. Their doctors were kind but helpless. When the battle was over, the sufferers on the field were taken on board the ships slowly and awkwardly, for want of the means by which our allies cleared the field of their wounded before the next sunrise; and it was the sailors who came ashore to offer help, and not the authorities on land who asked for assistance from the navy. There were transports in crowds, as well as the men-of-war: but no arrangements had been made for putting the sufferers into them. It was a sad sight,—the shipment of the wounded. It was better done henceforward. But contrary and impracticable orders made great confusion; and several vessels were overcrowded, while the supply of surgeons fell short. There was, indeed, plenty for them to do in the Crimea.

Ship Transport.—If the subject of organised hospitals and conveyance of the wounded had been entered upon in a business-like way, by consultation between military and medical authorities, there must have been an arrangement by which a certain proportion of vessels should have been fitted up for the conveyance of the sick from the seat of war to the hospital, or home. Each of those transports would have been a floating infirmary, supplied with surgeons, and with all means of sustaining the wounded during the passage. One main part of the arrangements would have been securing the speedy filling and immediate departure of each vessel; and another would have been employing the most orderly and quiet method of putting the sufferers on board at one end of the passage, and getting them into the hospital at the other. Very unlike this was the management at the outset. The painful scene on the beach, the day after the Alma, was one evidence of sheer unconsciousness of what was required. There were more evidences when sick were sent without notice to Scutari, so that they were longer on board, waiting to be landed, than they had been on the passage from the Crimea; and again, when ships were reported ready without notice, so that the sick could not be carried through the forms necessary for their removal, and the ships sailed without them; and again, when, in the autumn of 1855, a medical officer in the camp applied for transport to take the sick of his regiment down to

Balaclava, and saw them die before the means of conveyance were ready, a fortnight afterwards. The lesson of even the first few weeks was so clear that improvements were instituted by Christmas 1854. At that time, four ships were gradually fitted for the conveyance of the sick; and the transport agent did all that could be done to supply them with comforts.

Why the Quarter-master-general and the medical authorities did not arrange these matters between themselves and with the transport agent, and, on occasion, with the naval commanders, it is difficult to conceive; but it is safe to conclude that such a hitch can never occur again, if the people of England are as business-like as they are usually taken to be. The Quarter-master-general did intend to appoint an officer for the express duty of collecting the sick, and allotting them to ships about to sail: but the thing was never done. So the first who were carried on board lay tossing on the sea for days, while a few at a time were brought down; and it was an even chance whether the vessel would be overcrowded, or would start only half full, and whether there would not be another week to wait at the other end of the voyage. Three instances occurred in which the sick were on board three weeks: and they were seldom less than a week; whereas two or three days would have sufficed under a good established method, and the ordinary chances of weather. The mortality, always high among the sick so circumstanced, was fearfully aggravated by these delays. One vessel, "The Caduceus," freighted with cholera patients, carried 430, of whom 114 died in six days. When concert was established, this class of evils was overcome, with others. Meantime the story is one of the strongest admonitions ever addressed to human faculties to use those faculties in due consultation and arrangement before going to war. Consultation between the military and medical authorities, ensuring co-operation between the proper departments, may practically add no small proportion to the military strength of the country, simply by preserving that part of it which is in the field. For every soldier fairly allowed to recover, by the united wisdom of his military and medical superiors, a citizen remains at home, ready to be called out if his country wants him for its defence.

Need of Organisation. — Cholera and dysentery were still travelling with the troops when they reached the plateau before Sebastopol. What was done with the sick? The land and sea forces met at Balaclava on the 26th of September. From that time till the 19th of November there seems to have been no notion of putting them anywhere but into tents. During that interval we hear nothing of hospitals. The medical men could hardly have supposed that the force would remain long before Sebastopol. No doubt they expected it to be in the city, or away from it, very soon; and if so, this is another evidence of the mischief of reserves, involving life, between the commanders and the physicians of the troops. On the 26th of November, it was recommended to establish a General Hospital at Balaclava, repairing a building which would answer the purpose.

During the interval, it was a pitiable thing to be seized by the epidemic in that camp. Men were seen "wet, wearied, and half naked, borne by their comrades, or dragging themselves slowly and painfully along." Whither? To a tent, where they were at once breathing one another's breath, and quaking with cold. In a disease in which it is of extreme importance to keep up the natural warmth, the patients had no bedding, no blankets, no fuel; while their doctors received notice from the Purveyor to the Forces that there was "no arrow-root, brandy, essence of beef, sago, or candles, in store." Ground rice was again to serve for arrow-root; but it had not reached the camp from the ship, though repeatedly asked for. What could the doctors do in such a case? In October, the physicians complained that the men had had salt provisions for five days; and between the unwholesome food and want of tents more were falling ill every day. The tents could not be had; and the men were becoming scorbutic from other causes than salt provisions, — from want of fuel and cookery. Before the end of October, scurvy was reported to the Duke of Cambridge.

In November, the sick were still under bell tents, the hospital marquees being all the while on board the ships to which they were sent at Old Fort. The one thin blanket, and the need of more clothing and warmth, were so represented as to bring some Turkish mats and tarpaulins, — the latter apparently to sleep on, to avoid the wet ground. Orders were issued to cover up dung-heaps, and entreaties presented that horses might be picketed somewhere else than near hospital tents, and that rags and refuse might be swept up and burnt. The Balaclava hospital was overflowing presently after it was opened, and sick transport vessels were earnestly demanded to relieve the pressure.

By this time the state of affairs was appalling; but the authorities were arriving at some sort of notion of mutual concert, and of the benefit of seeking or accepting advice from each other. The departments, however, could not at once be rendered co-operative; so that more mischief must be endured before the retrieval could become apparent. On the 24th of November, 9003 of the nominal army of 37,232 were sick, — 2106 being present, and the rest absent. In other words, one-fourth of the army was sick. The fact was reported, not for the purpose of taking in hand so desperate a case, but simply because it was a pressing necessity to remove the burden from the camp. At this very time, — on that very day, — regiments were landed in heavy rain, and some of them were unsheltered, even by any kind of tent. This was a sign that the lowest point had not been reached; and a few more weeks proved it. The troops had met the enemy at Alma. They were meeting a worse foe before Sebastopol; but this foe is one that we have got under our foot. It is for the national wisdom and spirit to see that such ravage is never permitted again.

CHAP. V.

A WINTER IN CAMP.

Social Hygiene.—Many of my readers must remember the time when we, the people of England, were all quite free and easy as to where and how we would build our houses, and should have been exceedingly surprised if any person had interfered to find fault with any dwelling, or row of dwellings, that we had thought fit to erect for sale or hire. Many must remember not only the everlasting Irish cabin, with its dung-heap and pig, and its mud floor and its rotten thatch, but the brick cottages of English manufacturing towns, — rows of cottages run up on the clay soil, with little foundation and no drainage, with little windows that would not open in the front, and no windows at all at the back. Some of us used to fancy that it must be pleasant to live as the gipsies did, in a green lane, sleeping on the ground, with dew-dropping trees or hedges overhanging. Knowing nothing of the rheumatism and the fevers caused by grassy couches, and being smothered under a waggon tilt, we supposed such an open-air life to be something very fine. A group of cottages in a nook between hedges, or on a boggy bit of ground, — dwellings for men as dirty as birds' nests, and as airless as mouse-holes, and as damp as fungus-beds, were filled with labourers and their families as a matter of course; and any person who had proposed to examine the property, and to order that any improvements should be made, would have been supposed out of his senses. Gipsies might be meddled with as trespassers and vagrants; but if they had made a permanent lodging-house of their camp (the camp being on free soil) nobody would have dreamed of interposing, out of care for the health of the lodgers. We did not doubt, in those days, that any Englishman might build any number of castles, which nobody might enter but by his leave, — whether he lived in them himself or by proxy. It is not so very long since we began to admit that it was a social offence, and ought to be punishable as such, to build dwellings, or let lodgings in which it was impossible for the tenants to have their health. It is quite recently that we have become accustomed to the action of Officers of Health, when they examine premises, enforce the law against the makers of private bargains, (who fancied they had only themselves to please,) and publish the truth as to how many people die, and what they die of.

Recent as is this new kind of interference, it has been very well borne, on the whole. At the first glance this seems the most wonderful thing in the entire business. Most continental peoples are accustomed to have their affairs settled for them, and to see the police watching the whole economy of their lives; but Englishmen cannot endure the remotest approach to this management. Intrusion into their private affairs is resented with the force of an instinct in our country. Whence, then, the submission to sanitary officers, almost as thorough as submission to police vigilance in France or Austria?

The Englishman's reason is convinced; and hence his obedience. What is his reason convinced of? That the health of the public cannot be provided for by private arrangements only. This is one truth. Another is that the selfish interests of one person cannot justly be permitted to endanger the safety of many; and if the wrong cannot be kept in check but by the law and its agents, the law and its agents must be permitted to penetrate into the last recesses of the Englishman's property, — the damp cellar or mouldy garret of the lodging-house, — the cesspool on the one hand and the pigstye on the other. A sleepy citizen here and there may start at finding anybody daring to meddle with him and his property; but on the whole, the nation has responded very well to the call to admit of a new department of government, instituted to preserve life by a course of action too extensive for individual management.

Satisfactory as this is, we must remember how recent it is. Perhaps the first occasion on which we, as a people, became aware that a new department of social duty and welfare had been opened, was the first laying out of Birkenhead, — before the great suspension of operations which is now our chief association with the name and the place. To those who knew little of the methods of life among the Romans, it was very striking to see works equivalent to the building of a city, — extensive, elaborate, costly, laid out as mere preparation for the town which was to appear on the surface of the ground. The broad considerations of the soil and the air, and the water, all to be provided for before an inch of wall began to arise, were as impressive to the general public in one way as to unscrupulous speculative builders in another. Since that time, and since the contemporary inquiries by the Poor Law Board into the causes of the excessive mortality among the labouring population, we have risen to something like a practical notion of civil hygiene. We are aware that the health and life of persons living in society may be favoured and protected by securing good conditions of air, soil, water, dwellings, and food markets. Individuals must still take charge of their own health, as far as personal habits are concerned; but a great deal is necessary which individuals cannot do for themselves; and society — that is, the government — must undertake the management of these large conditions.

Military Hygiene. — If we were novices even thus far, when the late war began, it is not surprising that we were unprepared for the guardianship of the health of an army abroad. If civil hygiene was a new science and art to us, the more special art of military hygiene seems to have been unthought of, except in a desultory and ineffectual way, by an anxious official here and there. When the thing to be done was to set up an artificial city before Sebastopol, as Isabella of Spain established her host in an opposition town before Granada, no arrangements like those of Birkenhead were in question at all. Here was a population as large as that of our second-class towns, to be provided all at once with dwellings where there were no builders; with water where there were no companies or reservoirs; with food where there was no market; with clothes where there were no shops; with all the necessaries of life, in short, where there was nothing to be seen but the bare soil on a bleak table-land. "Hard conditions these!" it may be said. True; but they were the conditions of warfare, or the authorities thought they were; and that they were not fully considered, like other strategical arrangements, can be explained only by the general ignorance which had not yet taken warning from the loss of former armies.

The subject of the health of the army does not seem to have occurred to anybody, when the troops arrived before Sebastopol. A physician, who had appointed an Inspector to a particular division while at Varna, to see that nuisances were removed, and precautions taken, continued the practice before Sebastopol; but the Inspector soon died of fever incurred in the course of his work; and he seems to have been the only Health Officer till the alarm was taken, — too late. No sanitary council met, at the end of the march, to consult about making the camp healthy. No organisation was even proposed for seeing that the place was clean and wholesome, protecting the purity of the water, and keeping the soldiers warm, well fed, and well nursed. The liberality with which everything that could be thought of was supplied from England, shows what care would have been taken of our soldiers if it had been a recognised study to keep the army in health. Experience taught something at last; and in March 1855 a council was held on the subject of the health of the camp.

What do we now believe it possible and right to do in such a case?

The Soil.—It was some time before it was generally supposed in the camp that the army would remain there. Sebastopol might be taken before the winter set in. We all remember how confidently we hoped it, and how certainly the French Emperor expected it, when he was, like the rest of us, taken in by the false report that it was so. Great numbers of our soldiers probably hardly conceived of a winter on the plateau, till the desperate attempt of the Russians under General Liprandi, to dislodge us from Balaclava, had been foiled. The gallantry of that repulse was even more impressive to us at home than the battle of the Alma. It was no longer the first battle. Men knew better what the struggle was; and they were in even lower bodily condition. Scurvy was eating away their vigour; and cold and hunger were depressing the pulse and relaxing the nerve. Yet who could have thought it!

The enemy believed their way was clear when they saw the Turks flying from their batteries, and racing down into Balaclava; but in another moment, they saw the guns turned upon the recreant allies, and the British firmly planted to receive their charge down the slope, if they could not divert it by a timely fire. The British did so divert it, at a distance of fifty yards. They did hold their ground; they did keep Balaclava, and compel General Liprandi to account to his Emperor for failing to dislodge the besiegers. Our cavalry that day showed what the pluck of British soldiers may be under the most desperate circumstances. Worn by hardship before, misled by some unexplained mistake at the moment, sacrificed by one of the fatal accidents of the field, the cavalry who achieved the immortal Balaclava charge vindicated our character as a military nation for all time. Our troops afterwards heard the cheer with which the Sebastopol garrison and inhabitants received the false report of our having been driven away; they heard of the *Te Deum* being sung in the churches; and they were as undaunted as when they first set foot on that shore. Next day they were ready for the forces which came crowding up to see why they were not retiring from the siege; and that day they had matters all their own way. From this date, it seems to have been perceived that the plateau might be their home for more than the week or two talked of before General Liprandi came.

If there had been a sanitary council, therefore, it would have provided first for a short residence. Long or short, the first consideration is of the dryness and purity of the soil. Spades should have been at command to drain the sites of tents or other shelter; for there was plenty of rain, whether the soil was naturally wet or dry. The principles and practice of drainage being understood beforehand, the work should be as much a matter of course as pitching tents in rows, or setting up an impromptu bazaar, as the French do. A system of drains, simple and general, as far as circumstances permit, will hereafter be regarded as indispensable business, wherever troops stay long enough to admit of the process. As it happened, there was nothing of the sort done in this our day, even after huts had been sent out from England, and set up, and lived in. The first opinion we find on record, as to the causes of the sickness in camp, is on the 7th of December, when a medical officer represented that a certain regiment was suffering from exposure and damp. About a month later there were some huts up,—(though many more that were not) and the huts were as undrained as the tents or bare ground had been. "Undrained" is the complaint we meet with about the huts, for months after. Heavy rains flooded tents and everything in them.

The Air.—Next to the soil comes the air, though it used to be the custom to put it at the bottom of the list of essentials, if it was set down at all. The quantity and quality of air is the main condition of the life of every human being, though the commonness of the supply renders us careless of the fact. A proper sanitary department would provide for this, the very first hour of the ground being occupied. If the men sleep exposed, they have, of course, plenty of air. If they live in tents, they must not be allowed to heap earth round the outside so as to bank out the air, and then shut themselves in, however cold, without leaving any chink for bad air to be let out, and good to enter. We observe many complaints and orders about the earth heaped round the tents. It was damp, it grew foul, and it extinguished ventilation. After huts were provided, the men slept in them in considerable numbers, breathing together a very short allowance of air, while complaining of cold, and trying to get warm by shutting themselves up, and stopping every crevice they could get at. Several months after the huts were put up, we find, in the correspondence of the medical officers, recommendations that there should be turrets for ventilation in the roofs of the huts; holes bored in the planks, and so on. As to the quantity of air, we shall see more about it when we arrive at the subject of hospitals; but what can be done in a camp about its quality?

This is the grand consideration in regard to town life; and, indeed, we might say in regard to bodily life everywhere. Even nomade tribes, who inhabit the breezy desert or wilderness, are not necessarily supplied with a sufficiency of good air. My readers are probably acquainted with Mr. T. W. Atkinson's Siberian Travels, which tell of an open-air life of months and years, free and vigorous as the gales of the steppe themselves. What greater nuisance ever beset him than the foul air of the tents? What excited his pity so much as the disease, among the children particularly, which was the inevitable consequence of breathing such an atmosphere as the people slept in? The plateau before Sebastopol was sufficiently breezy, we should suppose; but, if the men shut out the air at night, they spoiled it by day. From page to page, we read of dead horses lying about. Under any kind of sanitary management that could not have happened. We consider it one of the barbarisms of the Red Indians, that the offal of fish and beasts litters their camps. It was on the 24th of January, 1855, that the first published suggestion is found, that dead animals should be buried, "instead of being allowed to decay, and taint the air above ground." Again and again we stumble on these dead animals, and on various other nuisances that one would think would almost cure themselves. It is requested, towards the end of the winter, that pioneers should be directed to clear away offal, dirt, rags, and condemned clothes from the neighbourhood of the hospital marquees and tents; and that horses may be stationed somewhere else than close by the sick tents. Any sanitary organisation would have rendered it impossible that the most robust soldier in camp should have been exposed to risks like this. The slightest knowledge and practice of military hygiene would have secured the regular clearing away of nuisances and rubbish, so as to preclude epidemics altogether. In all weathers and under all circumstances, that winter, it would have been good economy, good strategy, to have the camp regularly swept and purified. It might have been inconvenient; it might have been "impossible" (as the word is used), but if we had had the foresight of science, we should have found it a yet more impossible thing to sacrifice thousands of our best soldiers to foul air under the name of zymotic diseases. A twentieth part of the men who died needlessly in that way would have kept up cleanliness, and preserved the purity of the air, if we had understood as we do now the conditions of health in the artificial abode of the camp. It will never again be called impossible to consider first whether the site of a permanent camp be healthy, and then to keep it so. It might have been necessary to occupy the plateau before Sebastopol; but it was known, from works of travel and otherwise, to be unhealthy; and the question of its relation to the soldiers' health seems not to have been even stirred at all.

Personal Health.—As to the personal hygiene, it must be left to the medical officers to look after. The organisation which will, sooner or later, control the large conditions of the social health of cities or camps,—the organisation which keeps the site dry and clean, provides water for the wants of thousands by a machinery which supplies them all, and prevents the air being vitiated which a multitude is breathing at the same moment,—cannot look after the personal habits of individuals. It will still be the doctor's business to see that the men of his regiment do not stop up their breathing holes, as they are apt to do in barracks; that they observe personal cleanliness, and are properly clothed and fed, and that they are, if possible, saved from the temptation of poisonous drinks. In these duties the medical officers seem to have been exemplary during the last war. There is no mistaking the spirit in which many of them wrote and acted. It was no fault of theirs that the larger administration was never attempted at all. It was not their business. They undertook the charge of the sick, and to look to the health of the men under them individually. The care of the health of the army was not in their line. That it was in nobody's line was due to everybody's ignorance.

Nutrition.—Fuel.—The Quarter-Master-General's first care, we have seen, is about wood and water. It would have been that of a sanitary officer, after soil and air. It leads us to the consideration of the food-supply of the camp, and the actual nutrition of the soldiery. At the first glance, it may seem strange to treat under the same head of wood and water and food; but a moment's consideration will show how the supply of all relates to the same need. The bodily functions are feebly performed, and the body wears out under the depressing influences of cold and hunger: but, more than this, a portion of our food is actually the fuel of our frame: and again, that internal fuel cannot be properly supplied without the cookery for which external fuel is necessary. Food keeps us warm, on the one hand; and, on the other, the food which really nourishes must be cooked, and well cooked. No supply of wood in the camp would have kept the men warm in the absence of abundant food: and again, the largest supplies of food-stores could not keep them in health without the means of cooking their meals. A further instance of the dependence of one thing on another, in this kind of provision, appears in considering the water-supply of a camp. Unless there are sanitary guardians of the springs, the troops scramble for them; the strong party that gets possession of a spring-head spoils it by dipping so as to stir up the mud: more dirt is thrown in by the crowding; and good water is wasted by spilling, which again increases the mud. Horses scramble at the troughs; and if more troughs are added, one below another, to accommodate more horses, the lower portion of water runs to waste, because no horse will drink water that has passed the mouths of animals above. Under such management, the most copious spring is made to yield the smallest beneficial amount. Under proper sanitary authority the pure water would be economised, and the dirty cleansed. Every spring would be immediately boarded over, and a reservoir made and supplied with taps for the men's use (each tap yielding a pailful in five seconds), and with separate channels to a sufficiency of troughs for the animals. Gratings, with beds of charcoal and sand, would filter and rectify water which would otherwise be poisonous. Thus is wood wanted to preserve and purify water. Charcoal burning is an easy art, and one which should be understood by somebody or other in every army, as by every wandering body of men. In future, when a portable steam-engine, no more burdensome than a field-piece, is considered a necessary part of the equipment, boards, beams, and all forms of cut wood may be had, wherever wood grows, whether for the platforms of the artillery, or to cover in the water-springs, or make a reservoir for the greatest benefit of the greatest number. Under such methods a supply of fuel for the camp-cooking would be easier to obtain than it has ever been yet. Under the chance-medley system of which we may hope that the Crimea will have been the latest scene, our allies got possession of most of the springs, our soldiers had muddy or tainted water for all uses; and when the wells were spoiled, they were not repaired. As to fuel, we do not forget the narratives of wearied men from the trenches having to wander about pulling up bushes, or collecting any drift articles that would burn, and then to coax damp sticks to kindle, and get nothing but smoke, while their meal was yet uncooked, and there was no prospect of the water boiling. On the march, there were blazing bivouac fires, fed with broken furniture from the pretty villas and goodly farm-houses beside the road. Legs of tables, frames of mirrors, shelves and chair-backs made a grand fire to warm the weary; but in camp, when the poor fellows were yet more weary, and grievously worn and wasted, it was a less evil to go without the distasteful meal, or to eat it raw, than to labour at making the fire to cook it.

So much for the preliminaries to nutrition,—Wood and Water. As to nutrition itself, the days of the world's gross ignorance are past, and it seems impossible that any national soldiery can ever again be sacrificed to mistakes arising from that ignorance.

Old Rations.—When the rations for our troops

were fixed in 1813, and made in amount and quality very much like what they were for forty years after, there was little knowledge, even among professional men, of the precise uses and action of food. It was not so very long before that any accurate account could be given of the real process of feeding a fire; and there was great scoffing, only a dozen years earlier, at Sir Humphry Davy, and other philosophers, who recommended new and effective methods of nutrition of the soil, under the name of bone and other manures. At such a time it was not surprising that a philosopher who advised improved methods, on the same principles, of nourishing the animal frame was laughed at as a dreamer or an adventurer, till he proved his point by solid facts. Count Rumford's enterprise of feeding the Bavarian beggars could not be laughed down as a dream. The fact was too solid to be so blown away; but his doctrine that mere cooking, — mere boiling in water, — added a nutritious quality to food was ridiculed by our wise commonalty as the practice of boiling turnips for cattle is now, by old farm-labourers who "haw haw" on the village bench at the new fancies of their young masters. It was true, however, as Count Rumford said at the time, that the French prisoners at various stations in England contrived to live much better, — to swallow much more nourishment, — than labourers and others in their neighbourhood, who spent the same amount of money, or perhaps a good deal more, on nearly the same articles. The pence which the labourer's children, and the toiling labourer himself, consumed in the shape of dry bread, the French prisoner laid out in barley-meal, or pearl-barley, and red herring and a little bread; and fire and water did the rest. A thick stew, with balls of bread-crumbs and red herring cut fine, made a better meal than a round of bread; not only more palatable but more nutritious; but it was long before ignorant people could credit the fact. By 1813, therefore, we were by no means ready to look into the chemical and physiological merits of any proposed dietary; and, as forty years is a short period in the age of our institutions, that dietary was likely to exist without being subject to subversive remark till some such event occurred as the mortality in the Crimea. Such changes as were made in the management meantime rather excited the distrust of the soldier than improved his condition.

Sixpence was the stoppage from the soldier's pay in 1813; and his allowance was one pound of bread and three-quarters of a pound of meat. Twenty years later, an additional half-pound of bread was allotted to troops encamped in England. Abroad, the soldier had a quarter of a pound more meat, on the ground that foreign meat was inferior to English. Amidst many changes in the amount of stoppages, and in the administration of the food, the rule remained that a pound of bread (or three quarters of a pound of biscuit) and three-quarters of a pound of meat was sufficient food for a man in health. In point of fact, however, this would not do at all. The stoutest man will soon become diseased on such a diet. There must be some vegetables; and there ought to be considerable variety in food. Breakfast at half-past seven, and dinner at half-past twelve, were the two daily meals. It was not to be supposed that the men would pass the rest of the day in total abstinence. Some bought a sensible meal; but more spent their money in unwholesome ways, and especially in drink. An evening carouse, on an empty stomach, was bad for both health and morals; and some commanding officers introduced a remedy, some years ago, in the shape of a third daily meal, obtained by a stoppage agreed to by the men. The plan answered so well that it was extended to the whole army; and our soldiers became more healthy and more orderly. There was some power of choice as to what they would have at this meal, because it was managed by messes, the members of which had only themselves to please. The dinner was still boiled beef every day; and when the men got it baked out of barracks, they too often paid for the luxury of a baked dinner by diminishing their supply of vegetables. Such was the ordinary method at home, up to the beginning of the late war.

Rations in Camp.—When the army landed at

Varna, arrangements had been made to let the men buy from the Commissariat stores a variety of wholesome articles of food: but this lasted no longer than three weeks. Coffee and sugar were given out as a part of the regular ration;—but with this exception the men lived on their meat and bread. There were no markets at hand to provide anything else. This was a bad sign for the health of the troops when they should be encamped in a yet wilder place than the valley behind Varna. It was the business of one department to bring provisions in plenty to the spot, and of another to give out the rations: but there the arrangements stopped. It was assumed that the soldiers could not fail of being duly fed while the two departments did their work: but the men starved nevertheless. They did not understand the science of nourishing themselves, nor the art of cookery; and they suffered accordingly. The thing wanted was a department whose business it should be to see that every soldier actually had the command of a sufficiency of nutritious food every day. By good organisation this might be so managed as to constitute one part of the sanitary service of the camp. There is further ground of hope for the future, however, than even that of arrangements for every man obtaining his food in eatable condition. So much light is now thrown on the nature and uses of food, that the British soldier can hardly fail of being better nourished than he has ever been yet, and with a greater variety of food, at no cost of trouble or money, which can for a moment compare with the advantage.

The scientific facts which lie at the root of the new methods of army rations, which must ere long be adopted, are supplied by Dr. Christison, who was requested to make his observations on Sir John M'Neill's report on the soldiers' rations, and to propose a plan for feeding an army so as to keep the men in the best health.

Rationale of Food. — Dr. Christison tells us, in a popular way, what has been for some time familiarly known to physiological chemists, but has been, as he says, little imagined by "practical men." He tells us that nearly all our ordinary articles of diet contain some parts that are of no use for nourishment; such as water and an indigestible cellular tissue: — that the parts which nourish the body are of two classes: and that the most nutritious food of all is that which contains three parts of the one kind to one of the other. Thus, the best of all diets is that which contains the least of water and cellular tissue, and the nearest approach to the right proportion of the two sorts of nutritious substances.

How is it that there are two sorts of nutritious substances wanted? Because food answers two different purposes in the animal frame. One great use of food is to sustain respiration, which means to renew the blood, and keep all the functions active.

Another great use of food is to repair the waste which is continually going on in every part of the body, from the action of every part. The visible emaciation of starved persons is one sign and token of this waste: but it is not more true and serious than the wear and tear of every part, every day. Some portion of our food affords the material which goes to repair this waste; and the other part keeps up the action by which the material is conveyed to where it is wanted, and used for its proper purpose. The portion of our food which goes to support respiration and all that depends upon it, contains a great deal of carbon; and that class of nutritious substances is therefore called the *Carboniferous.* The other set,—that which goes to repair wasting substances,—always contains nitrogen; and that class is therefore called the *Nitrogenous.* Of these two, the nitrogenous sort is the most absolutely indispensable. Nothing can supply its place in repairing the waste of the parts of the frame: and without nitrogenous food therefore the man must die. Necessary as the carboniferous sort is for preserving full health, it can be done without, or a deficient quantity may keep a man alive, because the nitrogenous sort does, to a certain small extent, supply its place. Thus nitrogenous food is indispensable to life. Carboniferous food is indispensable to health, and to life in the long run, though its place may be in part supplied by the other sort of aliment. Again, the proper proportion of the two is one part (by weight) of the nitrogenous sort to three parts of the carboniferous.

In considering the quantity required to keep a man in health and vigour, it must be remembered that the weight of what he puts down his throat is a very different thing from the weight of actual nourishment contained in the food. The variations in the amount of refuse (water and innutritious substances) contained in different kinds of food are endless; and all that we have really to do with is the actual quantity of the two necessary elements mixed up with the rest.

Simple as this seems, now that we have been taught to regard food from the right point of view, it is a new idea of vast importance. Half a century ago, we were all as well satisfied as the most ignorant are now, that to eat a certain quantity every day is all that is necessary: that this is what the poor man should have; and that the luxury of rich men's tables is a mere tickling of the palate. That there was any third way we were not aware: — that, namely, of eating things which contain the greatest quantity of two particular elements with the smallest quantity of refuse, and so as to preserve the best proportion between those elements, care being taken to give the food in the manner most favourable for bringing out its value. It is true there were a few sayings which indicated some notion of the truth about food; but those sayings were very random, and often quite mistaken. "There is as much nourishment in an egg as in a pound of meat." That is one assertion, which is actually believed by some people at this day. There are thousands of even educated persons who suppose that chicken-broth and beef-tea are remarkably nourishing; and, though this is a mistake, the earnestness with which a teacupful is urged on a weak invalid, as including all the value of a full meal, shows some preparation for a real theory of food. So does the cottager's account of his pig-feeding; — of what he gives the animal "to stop the squeak," and what "to make bacon." These random notions were, however, a mere preparation for the great disclosure by which we see our way to the extinction of death by starvation, — at least, in our armies, — and to raising our soldiers to the highest condition of fitness for their noble work.

In ascertaining how much daily nourishment the health of the soldier requires, his mode of life is a main consideration. A clerk in a registry office, or a man committed to prison for a short term, cannot require so much nutrition as a hewer in a coal-pit, or a ploughman, or a fox-hunter. The prize-fighter is generally quoted as the consumer of the largest quantity of nourishment; and the weight set down for him is thirty-six ounces of pure nutrition per day. The copying clerk, and temporary prisoner, need only seventeen ounces, and are perhaps better with that than more. The soldier's wants vary with circumstances. Where the barrack life is (however tiresome) not an active one, he will not require more than men of average occupations; but when he is in the field, on the march, or encamped before a besieged town, sometimes fighting, sometimes working in the trenches, in all weathers, with much toil and disturbed rest, he needs almost the extreme amount of nutrition. Not only ought he to have it if he is to be kept in sufficient vigour for his business, and in spirits to meet the risks and hardships of war, but he must have it unless he is to perish. This is what we did not know in former wars. We grieved when our soldiers were underfed in any unfavourable turn of the fortunes of war. We would have given any money to feed them better; but we used to think, what I heard a clergyman say, in rebuke of forebodings about the harvest and the potato crops in 1845: "You know, nobody *does* die of scarcity." We supposed the want to be a temporary evil, and that the men would soon be growing strong again; whereas, we shall henceforth know, — if such a calamity as scarcity in the camp could ever happen again, — that the camp would certainly be half-emptied into the burial-ground, because the men would fall into a state of disease of one kind, while rendered unable to resist attacks of disease of any kind. The case is as clear as anything can be now that we understand it. We could always see that the waterwheel must slacken and stop when a drought dried up the stream. We felt the oven grow cool when the fire went down. We knew that, in like manner, people who had no food whatever must die within a certain time. But we did not always understand how the fowls in the poultry-yard became ragged and infested with vermin, and subject to swellings and flux, when a dishonest person stinted them in their food; nor did we know why our fruit-trees became a prey to all possible enemies and ailments, when we neglected to renew an impoverished soil. What we did perceive we never thought of applying to men in the aggregate.

We might call a sickly child "a sickly plant," and do our best to nourish it; but we did not regard a thronged city, or an army, as a forest of trees, whose vigour depends on their nutrition. I have seen in Kentucky woods where for miles there was scarcely a stunted plant, — the trees growing far enough apart for a carriage to pass everywhere, — the soil light and dry, and producing fine turf instead of rank weeds, and the verdure of each season lying thick about the roots, so as to manure every tree abundantly, and without intermission; so that the beeches and hollies spring to a height that we have no idea of in England, and nothing but our British oaks can compare with the Kentucky forest-trees in stability. I have also seen a forest in the Mississippi valley where the state of things was very different. Underwood and parasitical plants shrouded the whole space, so that the air was stagnant; rank weeds impoverished the soil; vermin pierced the bark, and corrupted the heart of many a tree: each one that fell left a slimy pool under its upturned root, and the poisonous water spread till it loosened the soil far and wide. Then, if a gale came from the east, after frolicking with the Kentucky giants, and doing them no harm in the playful wrestle, it had all its own way in the ill-fed and ill-ventilated forest. Down went every outward tree at the first stiff blow; and if the gale strengthened to a hurricane, the very heart of the forest was at its mercy. I have seen a wide gap through the very midst, where not a tree remained standing, but every one was snapped off at its weakest part. Thus was it with our force in the Crimea. Sapped by hardship, exhausted by want, infested with disease, when the epidemic came it laid everything low, felling thousands in their prime, and breaking them down at their weakest part. Now we know how it happened, may we not say that it can never happen again? We have only to say that it never must happen again.

Nothing could be further from everybody's thoughts than underfeeding the soldiers in the Crimea. We need not go over the painful history of the causes of the misfortune; and there is every reason why the notice of the state of the camp should be as short as possible.

Scurvy in the Camp.—The appearance of scurvy before the soldiers were made dependent on salt provisions surprised everybody. The men were, in fact, lowered in health and tone by what they had gone through in Bulgaria, and by damp and exposure since landing in the Crimea: and scurvy would have appeared, if there had not been an ounce of salt meat in store. The alarm was taken on the 17th of November: and by the end of December, more than half the infantry were sick in hospital,— the rate of mortality being higher than that of the great Plague of 1665 at its worst. A stir was immediately made to procure lime-juice,— from the authorities at home, from the Admiralty, from every naval station where it could be had. This was very right; but, as was said very sensibly, the soldiers could not live on lime-juice; and if they had had what was necessary to live on, there would have been little call for lime-juice. It must be added, that though a plentiful amount of it was sent at once, so as to be landed by the 20th of December, it was not used till Lord Raglan discovered its existence some weeks after. For five weeks the force was melting away in scurvy, and 20,000 pounds of the specific remedy was actually on shore, and it was never dispensed. After Lord Raglan found it out, the lime-juice was made a part of the daily ration, and was regularly served out from the beginning of February. At the very time that vegetables were a matter of life and death to the soldiers, a vast quantity of cabbages arrived at Balaclava, on the deck of a vessel. The captain could find no one who would take charge of them, or could suggest what should be done with them, and they were finally thrown into the sea because they would not keep. Preserved vegetables were offered to the men: but they had never seen any before,—could not easily believe that those little cakes could really be worth hungry men's attending to, and did not know how to cook them. These are the incidents which show us that it is not enough to send out plenty of stores, but that there must be somebody to take care that the men actually get what is intended for them, and that they then know how to use it. That in future the meals must either be supplied cooked, or the men be qualified or enabled to cook them, is a lesson which all parties have learned by a very painful experience.

The food they had seems to have been this:—

The Food.—The main part of the food was bread and meat, as it always is everywhere. But the bread was hard biscuit; and when scurvy tainted nearly the whole force, there were few of the men who could eat biscuit. The French manage to have soft bread wherever they go; and there is no reason why our troops should not, when the men have learned to bake. For some weeks there was fresh meat in turn with salt; and the quantity supposed and intended to be given was sixteen ounces per day, with a pound and a half of bread, or a pound of biscuit. But the salt meat was deceptive. Meat that is salted to keep two years requires so much soaking to get the salt out, that its gelatine and osmazôme are lost in the process, and much of its nutrition is gone. The plan of the men buying other articles for themselves broke down amidst such a scene as that of the siege of Sebastopol: the stores were distributed according to circumstances, and a portion of the pay regularly stopped for such supplies. In December we find that vegetables were issued at the rate of three-quarters of a pound for thirty-one days, or two potatoes and one onion daily per man, including the sick. In January the issue improved, being half a pound per week: and soon after preserved potatoes were to be had. The men cared more for rice than for almost any other article; and nothing could be better for them. There was a stock of 74,000 pounds at Balaclava, and four times as much at Scutari; and yet the two ounces per day, so precious to the men, was discontinued precisely at the time when they needed it most. Porter would have been in every way better than spirits, and there was a stock of it at Scutari unused, while our soldiers were toiling at Balaclava, sometimes without food for a whole day, and sure to swallow their grog the moment they could get it, from sheer exhaustion, without waiting to prepare the solid food. Sergeant Jowett tells us something about this in his truthful "Diary." He says, "Just fancy yourself in the middle of a field, up to your knees in snow, after walking about all night in it. You are hungry, and want something warm. Well, you have some raw coffee, some pork, and a little biscuit, with a small portion of sugar, and a little rum, or grog; of course you despatch the latter the moment you get hold of it. The other articles are different. You have no wood: none to be got, only the roots of brushwood. You manage to steal a pickaxe, for you cannot get one without, and then you commence grubbing for these roots. You are tired, but still you must have something warm. In the course of an hour or so, you manage to get a few roots; but the next thing is, how are you to light a fire? That has to be done, and must be done, if you wish to live. You manage to get your fire lighted after a great deal of trouble, and perhaps burning half the only shirt you have (that on your back), and then you have your raw coffee to roast or burn. You get a piece of tin, put the coffee berries on it, and place the tin over the fire. All this time perhaps you are almost frozen to death. When the berry gets black, put on your tin of water, and get a piece of an old sack that you have stolen from your employers, and two stones, and beat it to powder, and then wait till your water boils; you then put it into the water, and your coffee is made. You have then your pork to boil; but that is not much trouble after your fire is lighted. I wonder how many would like to pass away three months in the manner I just picture. Not many, I think, though strong." — *Diary of Sergeant William Jowett*, of the 7th Fusiliers, p. 47.

This is hardly the way to sustain the soldier's vigour, — or his spirit, — or his loyalty to the service; and this was the way the men got their meals for three months, as we see, while 147,000 gallons of porter were in store at Scutari, and 170,000 rations of tea were at Balaclava, and any quantity was obtainable in other directions. "We are in a miserable plight when we return to camp," says Jowett, "and perhaps for duty that night. Some days we get a quarter of a pound of pork, and about six ounces of biscuit. I am at this moment fit to eat my fingers' ends." This was on the 17th of December. About the beginning of February, two thousand coffee-mills were in camp, and fuel and roasted coffee were provided. Meantime, between the days when the men had all duty and no food, and the other days when they came off duty to feed in this way, the flower of our army were further from obtaining the needful amount of nutriment than pauper, gipsy, or thief at home. It was ignorance that did it. It would have cost incalculably less in every way — in trouble, time, money, and wear and tear of mind—to have had our soldiers marketed for, and cooked for, and served like companies of clerks and shopmen at home, with their hot legs of mutton, and steaming urns of coffee — than to lose and bury them. "I often wonder," says Jowett, sitting in the rain almost bare-foot, on a bundle of sticks (to keep *them* dry)— "I often wonder if a soldier will be treated the same in England as he used to be." Let us answer, "No;" —neither in England nor in any part of the world, now that we know what the soldier is, and how to take care of him. Now that we understand that there must be some authority charged with the care of the soldier's health, he can never again be so forlorn in the middle of the camp. Nobody at home knew, or could believe when told, that the British soldier could be so forlorn; nor was it credited within three miles of the spot. Parliament had granted money; Ministers had ordered that all comforts should abound; the War Office received accounts of the actual abundance despatched; and the commanders in the Crimea were assured that the stores had arrived at Balaclava, and were sufficient for everybody; yet we see how Sergeant Jowett was living. On the 10th of January, a grieving physician wrote to his commanding officer that the men were sinking for want of food. They got their food too late to cook it; no small time was necessary to prepare salt pork and unroasted coffee for the fire: the men had nothing to cook in but their camp kettles, which would boil but one thing at a time; or, at least, not salt pork and coffee: the greater number had not even the kettles, which they had been unable to carry, and were reduced to their mess-cans; and the poor fellows were actually eating the pork raw. Thus one thing hangs upon another. The men were sick at Varna, and therefore too weak to carry their kits, or even their kettles, in the Crimea; therefore they must cook in such a way that, to have coffee, it was difficult to boil the pork; and therefore the pork was often eaten raw. There was nobody in the Crimea, or anywhere else, whose business it was to see that the soldiers had their meals properly; and they had not been trained to do the best for themselves. The doctors could only recommend that more food should be given out — three meals a day; more rice, more vegetables, fresh meat daily, coffee ready roasted, and plenty of lime juice. What a difference between such a state of things and that in which scientific men are carefully estimating different vehicles of nutriment, and planning how best to make up the twenty-eight or thirty ounces of pure nourishment — twenty-one ounces of the one kind to seven of the other! To keep the men alive was more than could be hoped; and to keep them in health was a less reasonable expectation than to take Sebastopol within an hour.

The Wrong Methods. — The men had now tried the two ways of feeding — at home and abroad; the ways which were supposed inevitable, while we were yet in the dark about the principles of diet. Boiled beef every day in barracks at home, till the gorge rose at the sight of it, and the men sacrificed some of their vegetables to get a change; and in the camp, salt pork, half-soaked and half (or not at all) cooked; biscuit too hard for scurvy patients (and almost every man was scorbutic) to bite; and coffee in a yet more tantalizing state. These were the two wrong methods, belonging to a time of ignorance. We now know the right method, grounded upon knowledge.

The Right Method. — Taking the worst case first, that of an army on the march, or stationed where fresh provisions cannot be had at will, we now see, by Dr. Christison's help, why the men fail to eat their pound of salt beef or pork, when they actually need the nourishment it is supposed to contain. If duly soaked, it loses a good deal of that nourishment, and a different form of food is needed with it; therefore it is well to give four ounces less pork, with half a pint of peas (if in the shape of meal, so much the better), and, if the salt meat is beef, four ounces less of it, and flour and other materials for a pudding. This simple change would enable men to march further, and do and bear their duty better, by many degrees, than without it. Still, the inferior nutritive quality of salt meat renders the improved diet a very imperfect one; and the scientific certainty of this has caused an inquiry whether something better than salt meat cannot be had where fresh is out of the question. Great improvements can be introduced into the methods of preserving meat, in tins, in the form of pemmican, and, again, of meat-biscuit. The prejudices of the men against new articles of food cause a difficulty in adopting these inventions; but a very little instruction in cookery will alter their minds. When they discover that it is by getting rid of the water and other useless parts that the meat is brought into such small compass as the biscuit or the pemmican; and when they find what a soup grows under their own hands, from a few inches of the biscuit well stewed, with a few more inches of compressed vegetables, they cannot but be glad of such a change from salt pork daily. Fresh meat is better, of course; but the preserved meats, with rice, vegetables, or flour-puddings, may keep up the vigour of the men, if alternated with other forms of food. Wherever it is possible to take troops, it must be possible to take a kind of food so small in bulk as pemmican, which contains more nutriment than three times its weight of fresh meat. Under any circumstances, it may be well to provide meat-biscuit, because the materials are cooked in the making, and the biscuit may be eaten without further preparation. Instead of a man being "ready to eat his fingers' ends" at any moment, he can always be secured from excessive hunger by his ration of meat-biscuit. It is ready when he turns out suddenly in the morning; and it is a resource when he misses his meals, or has no time to boil his kettle. It would be worth more to him as a stew; but it is a meal of meat in any form.

The same may be said of cheese, which should be at command everywhere, if possible. "It is all nutriment," says Dr. Christison; therefore it occupies the smallest space. It keeps a considerable time with good management; and most men like it. Nothing but ignorance could have deprived our soldiers of such a resource in trying times. This is the unfavourable case,—of making war far away from home and its supplies. How will it be henceforth at home, or on a coast where our shipping can be the porters between home and the camp?

A New Dietary.—By putting sensible heads together a scheme has been made out which really seems to leave nothing to complain of. Military and civil officers, well acquainted with soldiers, have made out dietaries, to be pronounced upon by Dr. Christison in regard to the quantity and proportions of the nutritive substances they contain. The three meals per day proposed and pronounced on nearly attain the point of nutrition decided to be best, and certainly exceed, in quality and variety, any diet that the soldiers generally can have been accustomed to before they entered the service. Of course, their being underfed formerly is no reason for their being underfed as soldiers; but it is fair to rejoice in the removal of one of the difficulties in the way of recruiting our forces. It is a great gain to have got rid of the disrepute of the barrack diet, which it was known the soldiers loathed. It is a great gain to be able to offer to the young men of our army a mode of living at least as comfortable, in regard to food, as any they have ever known.

The breakfasts and suppers recommended are composed of coffee or cocoa (breakfast), and tea (supper) with sugar and milk, and eight ounces of bread: the sugar one ounce each meal, and the milk one gill; the coffee or cocoa one ounce, and the tea a quarter of an ounce. Of the dinners there are eight kinds,—a larger variety than is common in middle-class houses at home. Every dinner consists of a variety of articles,—meat and vegetables forming a part of each, with either pudding, bread, rice, or more than one sort of vegetables, and half a pint of beer. Beef, mutton, and pork, stewed, baked, or boiled; the vegetables, potatoes, greens, onions, and peas; the thickening, barley, rice, and pea-flour; the puddings, suet, batter, rice, and currant in variety,—this is an improvement on the daily boiled beef, which may go some way towards sustaining and replenishing the British army. Dr. Christison's translation of these meals into amounts of carboniferous and nitrogenous nutriment shows that very little is wanting to raise the diet to the point requisite for hard service.

But the cost?—Why, if the bread on certain days is exchanged for pudding (which would be preferred), there would still be a trifle left from the ration-money to get a little butter or cheese for breakfast or supper, with beer instead of tea. Further varieties might be devised by soldiers who knew how to set about preparing their food. What opportunities has the soldier of learning such things?

Camp Cookery. — It will never be forgotten that our allies had bread all through the campaign, while our poor fellows could not eat biscuit. We have learned, by hard experience, that bakehouses are as necessary a part of camps as any institution whatever. We have learned that such cooking-establishments as will save the waste and discomfort of every man preparing his own meals are a wise economy. A dozen men who by any means are enabled to have warm meals when they want them may be counted on for far better service than the same number who never know what a comfortable dinner is, and who do know, too well, what it is to be "fit to eat their own fingers' ends." We see and know these things now; but they must be provided for in time of peace; and therefore we were helpless when we made the discovery in the midst of war. Our allies had gone through the discipline before us, — in Algeria. There they had learned to shift for themselves, — to carry their *tentes d'abri;* to throw up a shelter against wind and snow; to obtain warm and agreeable food whenever it was in any way possible. Every Frenchman could cook, and certain numbers undertook the regular baking: while the British had had everything done for them, and had not had even the opportunity of learning how to take care of themselves. It will be a part of the soldiers' business henceforth to become able to shelter, warm, and feed themselves, under difficulties; and their friends will be greatly surprised if they do not like that part of their training, at least as well as any other. It is probably found at Aldershott, that the men have everything to learn; for the art of cookery has fallen very low among even women of the working class, — and indeed of all classes: but the art is not a difficult one; and when every man admits that health, vigour, and comfort depend on it, it is reasonable to require of the soldier that much exertion on his own behalf.

Practice at home will teach betimes what apparatus is necessary for preparing the meals of thousands of men. Thus far, the English soldier has had his mess-can, which he eats out of, and his camp-kettle, which does not hold water enough to cook a mess for five people, as it was expected to do. Just making a heap of roots or wood on the bare ground, open to all the winds, and then trying to boil his kettle, the soldier wasted as much as possible of the heat of his fire, the goodness of his food, and his own time and patience. More practised campaigners know the value of a sheltering bank, even if it be only a foot or two in height; and also of a trench so planned as that the air feeds without blowing the fire, and the heat is concentrated under the kettles. The example was not unnoticed, amidst the desolation of the first winter in the Crimea; and in January, and afterwards, as fast as the supply of kettles was renewed, our soldiers began to try to be more comfortable. It was the custom of the French to tell off ten men from each company to cook for the rest, which is more than necessary. In the British force very few could be spared; and when our men ceased to get wood and water, and prepare food each for himself, only two per company could be allowed for kitchen business. The kitchen was merely nominal. A fire was lighted behind a wall, if a wall could be had; and not even side walls of boards, or turf, or stones, seem to have been thought of, while the Turks (the best managers in the field), sheltered their fires and their kettles; and the French and Sardinians studied how to get the most comfort out of their means. The British so-called cooks had no idea how to set about their work. They had never been taught; and this was not the place for a lesson. Their main desire was to get out of the wind and rain in winter, and the sun in summer, as soon as possible. They did not know how to get the salt out of the meat; and there was nobody to teach, or even to superintend them. Here, again, we encounter the need of a Sanitary Department. The medical men could not be expected to interfere with the cooking. It was certainly no proper business of theirs. A few made strong remonstrances about the unwholesome quality of the food; but there was nobody to take it up. There was no Sanitary Department in the camp.

There was, however, a benefactor hovering about the destinies of our soldiers, in the shape of a cook, earnest in the cause of good and cheap nutrition: the late M. Soyer. He probably secured immortality to his name by connecting it with the rehabilitation of our army. We have lost him, with his zeal, and his knowledge, and his kindly regard for the welfare of the soldier and of everybody else; but we have his inventions; and we shall, I trust, put them to their full use. He proved that more nourishment is obtained from the combined rations of more than five than of fewer; while the saving from putting an end to individual cookery is enormous; and he proved that by his method, three-fourths of the fuel are saved, without any sacrifice under other heads. Considering the waste in cooking, the enormous expenditure of fuel, the loss and breakage and inconvenience of camp kettles, and the comparative discomfort, M. Soyer's Portable Boilers are pronounced economical in a pecuniary sense, while there is no doubt of their saving health and strength to an extent which cannot be measured by calculation. A mule carries two of these boilers, with sixty pounds of fuel; and the two will prepare the food of one hundred and twenty men; so that one mule per company, attended by the two men set apart for cooks, will abundantly serve. The soldiers will be spared the burden of their kettles, and will be sure of good meals; and all may learn cooking in turn, by serving as the second of the two men, — the first abiding as permanent cook. In ordinary marches and in camp the benefit will be great; and in forced marches soldiers carry neither kettles nor boilers, but rations ready cooked. There is no more difficulty about sending them boilers from home, and renewing them, than about the old camp kettles. It may be hoped that we shall never again hear of sickly and feeble men by hundreds throwing away their meat, because they can do nothing with it; and trying to live on biscuit which they cannot munch, and grog which injures an empty stomach, and turns a famished brain. Soyer's portable boilers supply good meat, vegetables and tea, when there is not fuel enough to light fires for a third of a company, besides sparing fires in summer altogether. Instead of the ten men per company appointed in the French camp, or even the two per company of the British camp, two cooks are enough for the whole regiment where Soyer's stoves are used. Water and stores being carried by fatigue-parties, two cooks can supply a good dinner to a thousand men. Twenty stoves in a row, — under cover, if possible, but quite effective in the open air, —attended by two men who understand their business, may save all the miserable fruitless struggles to get something eatable from hundreds of scanty, smoky fires, which are irritating the tempers of hundreds of cold and hungry men. Neither these stoves, nor any apparatus whatever, will serve men who are wholly ignorant of cooking; but if properly used, they may save a world of trouble and time, and (we need not fear to say) of health and life.

"Who will bake?" was the question sometimes, when there was at last a prospect of soft bread. "I will bake," says one, who has a fancy for a holiday. Some hours after, he is found drunk; a mass of heavy disgusting dough is drawn from the oven; and it is discovered that the fellow never baked in his life. Another kind of man says, on another occasion, that he will undertake the duty. He and some comrades have many a time scooped out an oven in the hill-side, or made a stove out of a trench and a few stones, with an iron hoop or two turned into a grating over the trench; and he finds it very easy work to provide a batch of light bread when he has an oven ready to his hand. The service of the stoves is therefore a matter of grave importance; and it appears that the best advisers recommend that, while all are recruited as soldiers, the particular abilities of the men should be utilised for the public service, and indulged for their own sake, as far as the circumstances of military life permit. Instead of attaching a certain number of non-military cooks to each regiment, it is recommended that the cooks should be soldiers who are skilled in the duty, and willing to undertake it. The rest should take it in turn to assist, to prevent undue dependence on the services of two or three. On such a plan the regiment may reckon on a daily meal, boiled, stewed, baked, or steamed; for Soyer's stoves will do everything but grill. Any one who has been up the Nile, or into the desert, knows how easily the thing may be done, when set about by practised people in a regular way. If a party of travellers in Arabia neglected to take a cook, and depended, as Californian emigrants do, on the kettle that swings and bangs about among the luggage, their fate would be much like that of our soldiers in the Crimea. We can fancy them on reaching their halting-place at the end of the day's journey,—not pierced with the cold, like Sergeant Jowett, but oppressed with heat, and drowsy and irritated with fatigue,—dispersing to get materials for their fire. Gathering thorns here, and digging up the roots of the white broom there, or making free with a wild palm, they may kindle a fire by the time they are too exhausted to stand. It is not a question of boiling there, where water is so precious,—unless the halt is by a spring; and the task of getting the mutton, or the fowl, rendered eatable, is so great a burden that, one after another, the party give it up, and eat whatever can be swallowed without cooking. The fire once being lighted, tea or coffee is a certain good for the evening; but to undergo the toil of a meal before starting in the morning would be too much; and biscuit and wine or other stimulant takes the place of the meat breakfast which desert travelling requires. This is not, however, the way in which we travel in Arabia. The portable kitchen, with its due supply of fuel, makes all easy. As soon as the tents are pitched, one of the native attendants is seen placing on the sand a little apparatus which is to work wonders;—two or three small iron troughs (according to the size of the dinner-party), with bars on one side, and an iron plate or set of bars to cover the top. As soon as the few inches of charcoal kindle, the stewing, baking, or grilling may begin; and in an hour and a half, or less, a luxurious meal is served. Soup, mutton, and fowls, in various forms from day to day, two or more kinds of vegetables, puddings, fruit pies, cheese and dessert,—such is the dinner sent up, hot and complete, from a kitchen of a yard or two square, if under cover, or open to the sky. In the morning, the red gleam of the charcoal shines before daylight; and, though the travellers are moving off in the dawn, they have enjoyed a meal of broiled or hashed mutton, fricasseed fowl, an omelet, dry toast, and tea or coffee. There seems to be no reason why twenty thousand soldiers on a march or in camp should not be fed in much the same way as twenty men and women travelling or halting in the desert. The provisions are there, the wood and water are assumed to be always there;—if stoves, with two men to attend on the cooking for a thousand, are there also, and are warranted to prepare excellent and varied meals, it seems as if that part of the soldier's trouble must be at an end. On the 28th of May, Sergeant Jowett wrote to his sister: "You cannot imagine how merry we all are; everything is comfortable in camp now." The people at home had helped to make this comfort. They had sent out everything they could think of in the way of food and clothing. Before the winter was quite gone, warm clothing was beginning to be served out, and huts to be set up. Vegetables, butter, and tea and sugar from England, were distributed on the 10th of March; and on the 24th of May, when the weather was, and had for weeks been, "hot and dry," the first draught of porter was enjoyed. Men were dying of cholera then, — generally from their own intemperance, Sergeant Jowett tells us; but neither he nor any one can tell how many of the victims fell into the habit from their dependence in the winter on the spirit ration for warmth, and forgetfulness of their hunger. The witnesses before the Army Sanitary Commission, who testify the most strongly against the spirit-ration, admit that it was necessary during the first dreadful winter in the Crimea. Never again should a poison become a necessary of life. A full diet, with coffee and tea, and porter in seasons of fatigue, may surely supersede the rum and grog. They were all actually in store when our soldiers were perishing. It was the administrative agency that was wanting. Even when a good road was made from the stores to the camp, and there was a Transport Corps to communicate between them, it did not follow that the men would be fed. There was still a chasm between the packages of clothes and the men's backs,—between the raw provisions and the men's mouths. A proper agency which should take care that the bales were opened, and the contents distributed—that the stoves were set up and at work—was still wanted as a safeguard against disease. The subject of camp cookery has been taken to heart: at Aldershott, ovens and ranges are erected in the huts; it is understood that the men are trained to make use of them: and the practice, once established, is not likely to be afterwards undervalued. But we have as yet no assurance that a sanitary agency will be organised for the army, express and extensive, so as to amount to a provision for the health of our soldiery corresponding with the provision for their sickness. We will presently consider what this agency ought to be.

Meantime, we must hasten over the other painful features of camp-life, as considered apart from the casualties of war.

Wants and Nuisances.—On the 2nd of December, says Sergeant Jowett, "one Jersey shirt" was served out to each man; but unfortunately it was only to each man of his own regiment. No boots were to be had that month; but the men comforted themselves with the thought that boots would have been but of little use in mud or water six or eight inches deep. The ragged boots and stockings were never pulled off, but disappeared piecemeal, as the men never undressed. If we are astonished at finding, by the professional correspondence, that the time and thoughts of medical officers were expended upon vermin poisons and small tooth combs, we cease to wonder at anything we meet when we open the diaries and letters of the soldiers. When his regiment was "nearly all gone," from death by dysentery, and the departure of survivors to hospital, Sergeant Jowett reports thus of himself:—"Thank God, I am quite well at present, having just recovered from a slight touch of bowel complaint, though not so well as when at home,—nor can I expect it, not having had my shoes or any of my clothes off for five months, but lying down every night, when not on duty, in full dress, with rifle by my side. I wonder what our sweethearts would think of us, if they were to see us now, unshaved, unwashed, and quite old men."—(P. 49.)

The entry "nothing particular" becomes very mournful as the winter gets on,—meaning the ordinary bad weather, disease and death. "Nothing more than usual to-day: (December 20th) that is, men dying very fast from dysentery and the severity of the weather." What was the rate of death which came to be considered "nothing particular,"—"nothing more than usual?"

Mortality.—The number of cases admitted into hospital in January alone was 11,290; and of these there died in hospital 3,168. Of this prodigious number of victims, all but 915 died of diseases caused by insufficient nutriment;—that is, of scurvy, and maladies of the scorbutic type. When we have once sustained such a calamity as the death of thousands of our soldiers in a single month from insufficient nourishment, we may well feel that we have had our lesson. But something more is necessary, as I have said, than resolving that a sufficiency of stores, of kitchens, and of cooks shall attend our armies wherever they move. The sanitary authority which is to be answerable for the men being nourished,—the means being provided,—is not yet in existence. It does not appear that its form and function, or indeed its very creation, have been determined on.

CHAP. VI.

PHYSICIANS, IN HEALTH AND DISEASE.

THE new knowledge that we possess about the causes of sickness justifies us in saying that the loss of an army by disease never need happen again. Our respect and regard for the British soldier impel us to say that it never shall happen again. To save our assertions from sinking into vain boasting, we must give our earnest attention to the method by which the health of the army may be effectually watched and guarded. What is the best scheme for a Sanitary Department of the army?

First Sanitary Movement.—The question occurs naturally in this place, because it was in the spring of 1855 that the idea of sanitary action occurred at once to various minds, and was presently acted upon. The army that went out was lost. Thousands of the men were in hospital, scattered through various countries. Thousands were sent home; and more thousands were under the sod. Fresh troops, sent to replace them, died even faster than the first army. We at home could not endure such a state of things; and one Commission was sent out to inquire into the supplies of the army, and another to devise and execute sanitary works for improving the health of the troops in the camp and in the hospital.

While both Commissions were on their way out, one of the surgeons in the Crimea called attention to the number of dead horses barely covered with earth in the Cavalry camp. He spoke so earnestly about the prospect of fever, that he obtained an inspection; and four camps were cleaned, and the dead animals properly buried. This was at the end of February. On the 6th of March, the two Commissions arrived at Constantinople; and the mail which would bring letters and notices of their errand was expected at Balaclava on the 8th; on which day it was suggested to Lord Raglan, by the chief medical officer on the spot, that a Board of Health should be appointed "to take into consideration the sanitary state of the army," in regard particularly to, 1st, diet and water; 2nd, accommodation for sick and well; 3rd, clothing; 4th, duty; 5th, locality. It will always be one of the strangest circumstances in our national recollection of the war, that whereas, first, the sanitary pioneers sent out before the war were snubbed and silenced, and that, next, there was no provision made for the sanitary charge of the forces, a Board of Health was proposed to sit in the vast grave-yard called the camp, after the army was lost, and after the Government at home had taken that business into its own hands. This, then, is the point of time at which it is natural to inquire by what management a due sanitary superintendence may be always ready to be applied anywhere, and under any circumstances, without room for dispute as to who is responsible for the health of the army.

Whose Business.—What should be done at the fountain-head,—the War Office? The military authorities in the War Office naturally pronounce that this is a business which belongs to the Army Medical Department. So be it, if it is understood that in future the entire subject of the physical welfare of the soldier is to be committed to army surgeons, specially trained for the work, and not that the doctors are necessarily sanitary officers, merely because they are doctors.

The Medical Department.—What is the Medical Department which is to take in hand this new branch of duty? Without going into the history of successive plans for the medical administration of the army, it is enough to say that the power and responsibility are vested in the Director-General of the Army Medical Department, who is assisted by Inspectors of Hospitals. The amount and variety of duties to be attended to by this chief officer might appal any man of sense and conscience who should be solicited to undertake them. He is responsible for the entire medical care of all our forces, amounting to 180,000 men, scattered to all parts of the world; and if he were more fortunate than any man has ever yet been in his subordinates, the charge is too heavy, because he is expected to know more, and to decide on more widely different affairs, than any one man can be supposed competent to. One consequence is that the Director-General is in constant need of counsel. He lays hold of every medical man who comes within reach, to get not only information but an opinion from him. Depending for counsel on the accidental neighbourhood of physicians qualified to advise, and assisted by clerks as to the multifarious business of his office, the Director-General ought rather to be largely relieved of his existing weight of cares than loaded with the responsibilities and toils of a new function. This will hardly be questioned by any one.

Its Reconstitution.—The Sanitary Commissioners seem to have been strongly impressed with the urgent need of a reconstitution of the Medical Department altogether. The nation certainly expects that a Department which conspicuously failed in its charge of the sick, in spite of the exemplary devotedness of the individuals of the profession, should be rendered equal to its duty before another war; which can be done only by reorganising it, and putting it on trial in a time of peace. The recommendations of the Commissioners are simple, and worthy of all deference and support.

The Director-General. — The Director-General ought to retain the power of acting on his own opinion, after having obtained the advice of his council. Where the authority and responsibility are divided, there are sure to be jealousies and quarrels, and an omission of some part or other of the business. Where the authority and responsibility are vested in a Board, the public interest gives way to the convenience of the members, who can hold together only by compromises. A responsible *chef* seems indispensable. But he must not be required to form decisions without being properly supplied with materials for a judgment. However able and informed a man he may be, he cannot be the very ablest in several departments at once. He must need the best counsel that can be had on medical and surgical administration, and on sanitary business, and on that department which requires a different kind of ability and knowledge, while it is as necessary as any other,—the physical statistics of the army. It is, therefore, recommended that the Director-General shall have a council consisting of three members, selected for their eminence in medical, sanitary, and statistical knowledge, and appointed by the Secretary for War.

His Council.—These counsellors would be charged with attending to the routine business of their several departments; and when any questions or considerations of importance occurred to them, they would submit them to the Council, and give their opinions in writing,—their judgment being always at the service of the Director-General. All the proceedings at the Board would be recorded by the secretary; and, if the *chef* should decide contrary to the opinions of his Council, he would record his reasons in writing. The details will be discussed to more effect in another place than this; such as the term of office in each case, and the amount of salary. The urgent point is to get the Council established, and the method put in exercise without any delay, that we may never again be found unprepared to protect our army from disease, in the field abroad, or in barracks at home.

So much for the fountain-head. How is the sanitary duty to be distributed?

Sanitary Officers in the Army.—Wherever there is an extensive assemblage of soldiers, sick or well, there should be a functionary charged with the duty of making their position and circumstances as wholesome as possible. Of hospital management, I shall have to speak further on. As to camps, or the quartering of troops in towns in war-time, it is proposed that there should always be a Sanitary officer attached to the Quarter-Master-General's Department, the head of a sanitary police, to recommend such measures as are needed to render the men's abodes safe, and their food and clothing appropriate to their wants; the military authorities being charged with the responsibility of accepting or rejecting his advice. He will be required to afford a judgment of the spot proposed for a camp, and to point out what should be done to make town quarters fit for human habitation. But there would be little use in this, unless some one were made responsible for carrying out his recommendations.

In the same way, if the men needed change of clothing from change of season, or alterations in their food, he must be enabled to give similar advice, under similar conditions as to execution. It would be an immense relief to the military authorities, one would think, to have a set of men with them whose business it is to see to the proper sheltering, feeding and clothing, and airing and watering of the force; and the Quarter-Master-General, above all, must be glad to commit to a qualified person the considerations, to him so confused and obscure and anxious, of the hygienic character of the preparations for settling the soldiers.

State of Balaclava.—The case of Balaclava was very striking. The town contained between 500 and 600 inhabitants before the army appeared above it. Sergeant Jowett was delighted with the first view of it. "A prettier little valley I never saw in my life; fruit in abundance; in fact, everything we could wish for. The poor people had all run away, and left their homes; they appeared to be quite taken by surprise." By other testimony, the place was as neat as a Dutch town. If the army had been supplied with sanitary officers, the valley would have been put in order for the coming crowd, and secured from corruption, before the men were allowed to enter upon any other business. A few hours at first would have made wharfs, and secured the watercourses, and made provision for the interment of dead bodies and other corrupting substances, and cleaned the dwellings, and arranged for the regular clearance of the harbour from all floating refuse. As there was nobody to do the preventive part, all the efforts of the Commandant and the Admiral failed to cure the mischief at a later time.

When at length the Board of Health was proposed, in March, 1855, the east side of the harbour had long been one mass of putrescence. Animals and vegetables had been thrown away there, and the salt waters passed through the refuse on the shore, causing an intolerable stench, and floated the blown carcases of dead horses and decayed vegetables. At the head of the little harbour, the burying-ground was to the last degree offensive. I will not describe it. Now, if preventive methods had been instituted here, decency, and even health, might have been preserved, though 30,000 men were crowded where five or six hundred had lived before. A sanitary police would have prevented the killing of animals elsewhere than in the place of slaughter, and would have seen the offal buried; and so on throughout. When the road was made, and the best cleansing effected that the military and naval authorities could order, the state of things was far inferior to what prevention would have made it; and in the interval, thousands of men had died. Cholera and fever broke out, again and again, in the town and in the shipping in the harbour, between May and September; and Admiral Boxer himself fell a victim to cholera in June.

But Balaclava became healthy at last, and while the crowd was still there. How was it? The Sanitary Commission undertook at last the business that should have been done first. Whatever filth could be burnt was burnt. The rest was, if moveable, carried out far to sea and sunk; if not moveable (as the contents of the graveyard) it was thickly covered with lime, charcoal, and earth. Each dirty office had its proper place appointed, and the refuse disposed of. The decaying matter on the east side was deodorised and covered in; the shoal water at the head of the harbour was made dry land; the worst houses were pulled down, and the others cleaned and whitewashed within and without; drains were made, and stenches disappeared; the ships were cleansed, and daily surveyed by three naval surgeons, who acted as a sanitary police. So many had died, that the work went on slowly for want of hands; but by July the worst was over, and in a few weeks more "Balaclava became what it might have been from the beginning, as healthy a little seaport as can be seen."

I must add a similar illustration from the camp

above. In the same spring, Sir Colin Campbell was unhappy about a portion of his brigade who were ill with fever in huts which appeared to be in a healthy situation on the heights north-east of Balaclava. The General spoke to the Sanitary Commissioners about it, and they examined the spot. They declared that the cause must be local, and advised the removal of the men. The General had a board taken up in one of the floors, and thrust down his cane into the soft ooze which was found beneath; it came up stinking. Under the eye of a sanitary police, the huts would never have been erected as they were, with one-fourth of each inserted into the hill, so as to intercept the drainage from above, which settled below and reeked into the huts when the men's bodies warmed the floor as they slept, just two inches above the surface of the ooze. The warm damp caused the fever. As soon as the inmates were removed to tents higher up, the sick recovered, and there was no more fever. I wish this was the end of the story: but there is a terrible sequel. A month later, that is, in May, 1855, a newly-arrived regiment was put into the empty huts which stood convenient; cholera broke out among them, and when thirty-four had died, the rest were marched to the front: but they could not leave the cholera in the huts, though they had caught it there; and seventeen more died. The huts stood empty then till November, when four companies of the Royal Artillery were landed and brought to them, three companies being quartered in the huts, and the fourth close at hand. Seven men in the huts died of cholera; but of the company outside not one. The same huts were removed to fresh ground higher up; and only one more cholera patient died. If there had been a Sanitary Department, with its police on the spot, those huts would have been properly placed from the first; and all this sickness, and death, and diminution of force, and sorrow, and remorse would have been spared.

Immediate Steps.—The necessity of a Sanitary Department in the management of the army being by this time pretty evident, the next consideration is how to set about putting it into action.

Sanitary Councillor.—It may not be possible to fill up in a moment the place at the Council-board appropriate to the sanitary member. It would be better to wait a little than not to obtain the best man; and while there are few who would think of pretending to adequate knowledge in Civil Hygiene, there can hardly be any who have even studied Military Hygiene with any completeness. In a future chapter I shall have occasion to show how unreliable are the bases of the calculations and reports of the best-intentioned inquirers in the civil department of the study, and there is no saying when a man may be found competent to the charge of the military branch. Any genuine student of the science and art, who is at the same time a man of sense and cultivation, would be a treasure at the Council-board, if the alternative were the subject being neglected; but we must have a better option than that. It must be a settled matter that the place is to be filled; and that made sure, we had better take time to ascertain the best man, than begin in a hurry at that particular part of the business, while there are other ways of being active upon it.

Reform.—Among those other ways, the most important perhaps is carrying out a thorough sanitary reform in our military institutions at home and in our dependencies, as has been begun by a Commission for improving barracks and hospitals, of which Mr. Sidney Herbert is chairman. Every barrack, camp, garrison, and hospital should be examined, and rendered healthy, according to the best existing knowledge. It would be folly to object to the cost, clear as the evidence is that the death and invaliding of soldiers is far more costly than any possible expenditure for sanitary purposes; but in fact, a prodigious amount of improvement may be carried out at a moderate expense. There seems to be no reason why this regeneration of the abodes of the soldiers, and also of their modes of diet and clothing, should be delayed for a single day. What we hear from India of the effects of the earliest acts of reform is very encouraging. Nowhere was barrack reform so urgently needed, and nowhere can it be received more gratefully. Instead of Dumdum barracks, where five hundred women and children out of a thousand died of bad air in fifteen months, we hear now of such barracks as Sir Charles Napier demanded for the soldiers: and the soldiers do not forget who demanded them. Instead of calling their new quarters by the names belonging to different localities, they call them all "Napier barracks," giving the humane old General one more hold on immortality.

From India we hear, too, of that reform in the clothing of the troops, which ought to be going on whether the seat at the Council-board is filled or waiting for an occupant. From Bengal we learn that the stock is abolished. It will be an eternal wonder why that murderous article of dress was ever worn again after the occurrence of one case of apoplexy clearly ascribable to its use. A century of scarlet coats, heavy or metal head-gear, and leathern stocks, in the climate of India, has been as murderous as many a cruel foe; but, at last, we hear of light and white head coverings, a loose, cool dun-coloured dress, and uncompressed throats. Such a change as this, with airy, well-drained barracks, and drill in the cool hours, must alter the conditions of the soldier's life in India beyond all calculation. Throughout the empire there should be a thorough rectification of all regulations which involve the soldier's health. In every department, the Quartermaster-General's, the Purveyor's, and those of hospitals and barracks, the regulations should be revised for the purpose of rendering them as conducive to health as they can be made.

A Sanitary School. — One other procedure may as well be going on: — the training in a Hygienic School. The chief reason why the French fared so much better than our troops at the outset of the Crimean war was, that their medical officers had been specially instructed in military hygiene in preparation for service. If it should be imagined by any reader that our army physicians must have had the same knowledge, though they did not give pompous names to it, the notion, however natural, would give way at once within the doors of such a school as we ought to have. The mere sight of the models, maps, and other apparatus, would show that this is a kind of knowledge which does not come of itself, nor in the company of medical knowledge. The requisite amount of geological study is not small; for it is necessary to know what diseases are likely to arise from settlements on all the various kinds of soil and sub-soils, affecting as they do the water, the natural drainage, the atmosphere, and, in short, almost all the conditions of physical life to those living upon them. Then, the student must learn to track mischievous agents through their whole action, — to find them in the air, and the water, and the food, and in many forms of disease. He must know the effects and liabilities of every kind of shelter overhead, as well as of ground underfoot; — the tent, the hut, the town flat roof, and the village loft; — the hot slates, thin canvas, damp thatch, and dirty clay, having each its dangers. He must understand the science and art of ventilation, as not one man in a hundred thousand understands it yet. He must acquire a knowledge of the principles on which works are carried out by sanitary engineers in civil life, and must add to it whatever is known of the conditions of health in foreign countries. He must learn what diseases prevail in each region; and why; and how they can best be met in the case of a camp population. He must learn all the special liabilities of camp life, and be familiar with the causes and control of epidemics. He must know the hygienic effects of all diets in all countries and climates, and must have the chemical science and skill necessary for ascertaining with quickness and certainty the composition and adulteration of whatever the soldiers swallow or breathe. He must understand the effects of all kinds of professional exercise and duty on health, and of all methods of clothing and warming the troops. He must understand the treatment of food and water, so as to secure for the soldiers, and especially for those in hospital, the best nourishment that the material will yield. These are a portion of the studies indispensable to any intelligent government of the physical affairs of an army. There has been hitherto no medical or other school to which any military or medical student could apply for means of instruction in these branches of knowledge. Henceforth there must be such a school. At any cost it would be cheap; but it need not be costly. The sanitary function once expressly recognised in the army organisation, and a body of trained scientific and practical men being secured to the service, the military officials would not only treat them with respect, but would be truly and heartily glad of their presence. Commanding officers would be relieved of a great weight of care from the hour when they could rely upon the health of their troops being guarded from the consequences of their own ignorance of a science which they could not be expected to study. Once supply the army with men competent, amongst other things, to undertake the duties of health-officers, and they will be abundantly consulted and made use of.

Question of a separate Department.—Who are these officers to be? Through our life-long association of the idea of physicians and surgeons with the actual ills of the body, we naturally think of medical men as our proper guardians against its possible ills; but the medical man is no wiser than other men about the agencies which endanger the healthy body, unless he has made them his special study. Our medical men have not done this, — not having had the opportunity. They understand the structure of the healthy human body, and its changes of structure in organic disease. They have learned what is known of the action of the organs of the body, in health and disease; and it is their special study and art to rectify what is wrong in that action. All this is something quite different from knowing what influences act injuriously on health, and practically precluding those influences. As an illustration of the case we have the fact that nothing has ever been done in the way of sanitary improvement by all the medical men in England. Till sanitary officers introduced the science and the art, fevers ran their course, and infested our towns, from century to century. The same thing was seen in the smaller field of the Crimea. Anxious and devoted as were the individual surgeons, and strongly as a few of them complained of filth and stenches, no sanitary management and method were proposed by the medical authorities till the Commissioners sent out from England had arrived at Constantinople, on their way to the camp.

But is this a reason why the medical and sanitary departments should not be united? That is a point for very careful consideration; and such consideration has been given to it by the sub-committee appointed for the purpose by the Royal Sanitary Commission. Here are some of the points involved.

The existing Medical Department is unqualified. About that there will be no dispute. The professional body cannot go to school again, to study a new branch of knowledge. We must then have a new body of officials. The real question is — shall we have a greater number of new medical officers, educated for both branches of practice? or shall we have a medical body of the usual proportions, and a smaller one of sanitary officers? Is there any advantage in the new ones being medical men? Have not the doctors quite enough on their hands in the care of disease, without undertaking the care of health? Why join two different professions in this particular case when we do not think of it in any other? These are some of the questions which require an answer. Something very like an answer is found in the indisputable truth that, in science and art, every specialty requires an unlimited, and therefore unmixed devotion of the faculties. Each of these branches of study is a specialty: each requires the unmingled application of the mind. Where, then, is the wisdom of requiring from any one man proficiency in both? If there is any objection to this view, it probably arises out of an inability to believe that sanitary science is so special and so extensive a kind of knowledge as is represented. In the course of another chapter or two, some light may be thrown upon the nature and extent of this field of study.

If we allow the popular impression to prevail that we have a right to require of our army-doctors the preservation of the health of the army, and end by charging the Medical Department with the hygienic office in addition to its own, we must not only strengthen, to a considerable degree, the force of the department, but alter the plan of its education.

Special Medical Education. — Army medical officers ought to have, if they have not, an education considerably different from that of medical civilians. As far as ordinary diseases go, and the casualties which occur in civil life, the preparation may be the same in both. A case of inflammation or indigestion may be just the same in London and before Sebastopol, and so may the act of amputating a limb; but the general character of practice is different. The army medical officer has to deal with the diseases of a vast body of men, living under unusual conditions, and subject to sweeping attacks of epidemics, and to a large amount of disease under a very few heads. He prepares himself, or ought to prepare himself, to deal with injuries which are seldom met with in civil life. Gunshot wounds afford, we are told, a wide field of study. How is this difference between civil and military practice actually met?

Candidates for the army medical service present themselves for examination, producing certificates of their having gone through the course of study which enables civilians to enter upon practice. They are, in fact, civilians applying for admission to military practice. The certificates may or may not testify to medical studies having been pursued, as well as surgical. The examiners are appointed by the same person who names the candidates; some inquire about one thing, and some about another; the questions (about forty) test nothing; but when they are got through, the candidate may prepare for the military field of practice, in which he is to pass his life. How is this done? He is sent to Chatham — to the Invalid Depôt at Fort Pitt, and to the General Hospital at Chatham. What to learn? Why, exactly what he has just been certified to know. There is no special instruction to be had there; or, till very recently, there was not; for it is only in consequence of the Commissioners' report that Government has granted an embryo school of the needed kind, at Chatham. The student may be there a week, or he may be there a year. He waits till there is a vacancy for him. Once posted, his destiny becomes serious enough. The young military officer, entering on service, is at the bottom of a set of twenty or thirty officers, and has time to learn and practice his profession by degrees; but the medical officer has only one or two seniors interposing between him and a tremendous responsibility, which any one of a multitude of chances may devolve upon him at any hour. This is hardly the process by which medical men can be duly prepared for the business of treating disease and bodily injury on a great scale. Shall the care of the army's health be added? It cannot, without some essential changes.

This is not the place for speaking of the hospital training of army physicians and surgeons. I need only direct attention to the need of a special training, supplementary to that held in common with the civil department of the profession. But this is the place for saying that, if the sanitary care of the army is to be consigned to the Medical Department, a special education in the sanitary school must also be required.

Conditions of Amalgamation.—This seems a great deal to demand of the members of any profession. What do the Commissioners think of the possibility of devolving on the Medical Department the sanitary charge of the army? They think it may be done on two conditions; that the Director-General has a sanitary adviser at his Council-board; and that the best possible medical and sanitary schools are provided, and fully made use of by every medical man who enters the service of the army. On these conditions the thing may be done: but the question remains, whether there are not preponderant reasons for keeping apart two services which are essentially distinct.

CHAP. VII.

THE WOUNDED AND SICK.

THUS far, I have said scarcely a word of the enemy in Sebastopol,—or indeed of any state of war in which our soldiers were living and dying. The calamities of sickness were in fact so much more fatal, and even more conspicuous, than those of the mere strife with the Russians that, without affectation, they occupy our attention now, almost to the exclusion of the incidents of the siege and the battle-field. We ought not to forget, however, that during the winter we have been dwelling on, the vast stores of ammunition collected in Sebastopol were poured out on our forces, like an ever-recurring hailstorm of iron and fire. When the din ceased, men thought themselves deaf,—so unnatural was the comparative stillness of that group of camps, and hum of tens of thousands of manly voices, which in fact resounded like a city. Every man saw wounds and death perhaps every day. Every man expected wounds or death almost every day. It is nothing new or surprising to say that there was no quailing in the midst of such a life, prolonged as it was from week to week, and from month to month. We cannot conceive of the British soldier as quailing under the liabilities he went out to meet. Yet, we ought to consider what the liability amounted to, not only because we are contemplating the life of the army, but because the resistance of Sebastopol transcends everything known in history for the deadliness of the destruction attempted.

Service in the Trenches —Life in the trenches was life face to face with death. Shot and shell hurtled without ceasing; and escape seemed more wonderful than any amount of slaughter. In those trenches, however, the martial spirit glowed, like their fires in a frosty night, and bade defiance to the chill dread of death. There the men listened with all their souls to any one who could speak from knowledge of the great wars under Wellington, and above all, to passages recited from Sir W. Napier's "History of the Peninsular War." When the shot came, the fortune of war was accepted gallantly; and the long-drawn pains and penalties were endured with a stout, simple, silent fortitude, more moving in the contemplation than even the preparatory valour. Sergeant Jowett spoke the sense of the army generally when he wrote to his sister a cheerful remonstrance against her anxiety about his days and nights in the trenches: "Think, my dear girl, the cause we are fighting for is *liberty*—which is dearer than life to any true-bred Englishman." But there was something finer than even all this. The men faced suffering and death by the most abhorrent disease as gallantly as in the heat of conflict. Each was thankful when any comrade was favoured with the nobler death (as they considered it); yet each seemed able to endure the apparently ignoble and disgusting lot of dying like rotten sheep. Here was the highest heroism. Here was the test of the soldierly character being ingrained in the very nature of our men; and we must acknowledge it with emphasis, and record it with clearness and diligence, because it must be our last opportunity. It rests with the people of England to resolve that their soldiers shall never more die like rotten sheep. We now know how to protect them from a destruction more fatal than all the ammunition in Sebastopol could inflict; and we must do them the justice to take care that their heroism has every enjoyment of its own mood,—that the flesh shall be as strong as the spirit is high.

On the Battle-Field.—When the scenery of the trenches was new to our imaginations, it naturally occupied them to the exclusion of yet graver subjects. The letters from the camp abounded in the details of military duty, while little was said (by soldiers) of the epidemic which was at the moment becoming like the Great Plague of London in its worst stage. When we learned the truth, it was not from the soldiers, nor from any complaining victims, but from intrepid champions of the soldiery. This is a reason why we should now remember the more emphatically that the great deeds of valour in the field were done by men worn with fatigue and hunger, and enfeebled by sickness. A battle was fought which is, and ever will be, called "the Soldiers' Battle," because circumstances prevented their commanders from using the ordinary foresight and control, and the men achieved the victory by their own force: yet the men who put out that force, and sustained it through a conflict of eight hours, were for the most part hungry, weary, and weakened by sickness and want.—Thus we find ourselves brought round to the same dreary view, from whatever point we start. We may set our faces towards the city, or the trenches, or the out-lying pickets, or the thick of the fight; but we find ourselves at last in the tents where the men are dying fastest and most drearily,—of dysentery, fever, or cholera.

Inkerman.—Yet we must not forget the martial part of the experience. Above all, we must cherish the memory, and all the traditions, of the November day which opened mysteriously to the men in the foremost trenches.—At one in the morning they heard the tolling of a church bell, faintly but continuously; and, at intervals, something like the swell of church music. By degrees other bells joined in, till every listener said there must be some remarkable observance going on;—probably some great saint's day of the Greek Church. No one of them suspected what was coming. The arrival of reinforcements on the north side of the city had been observed: it was known that a vast strength of men and stores had been poured into Sebastopol since the battle of Balaclava; but this and the tolling of the bells was not at once connected in the listeners' minds. That 5th of November was indeed set apart for a great religious observance,—for a crusade against the enemies of the popular church. Deserters and escaped prisoners and country people had told in Sebastopol how some churches in Balaclava were used for other purposes than the Greek worship; and this seems to have roused to the utmost the fanaticism which had treated this as a religious war from the beginning; and throughout the Russian empire it seems to have been resolved that this day would, by the aid of the saints, decide the fortune of the war. Prince Menschikoff had written to the Emperor his request that two of the princes should be present, to witness the defeat and humiliation of the enemy; and they were sent accordingly. Fifty thousand men were appointed and prepared for the holy fight. That night, all Sebastopol was awake, and at its devotions in the churches. It was a festival night, as well as a devout one. No one doubted that before the next noon the allies would be driven into the sea; and thanks were returned, and the brave were celebrated in advance. The troops were well fed, and plied with drink, so as to exalt their passions to a high pitch. The testimony to this fact on the particular occasion of the battle of Inkerman is so various and so strong as to leave no doubt that stimulating the men with brandy was one of the chief preparations. Thus passed the night in the city,—amidst lights and psalmody, bells and processions, feasts and imperial speeches, devotion and patriotic confidence.

How was it on the heights above? The pickets of the allies could see nothing, because a thick fog had settled on all the high grounds, and besides, it was a wet night. A drizzling rain, lasting all night, turned to a heavier down-pour towards day-break. Of the men in the foremost lines, some who were in too comfortless a state to sleep remarked on the sounds from below, to which was now added the dull rumble of artillery, not yet recognised. Behind, those slept who could; and some rose early to set about the arduous work of procuring breakfast. Some on the right were entirely absorbed in the effort to kindle fires, in spite of the rain, to cook their breakfast, without having any idea of being watched from behind the curtain of mist which enclosed them. Something greyer than the mist was observed by somebody to be in motion below it: and the cry "Here are the Russians!" made every man spring to his feet, and snatch his arms. The next moment up came the Russian heads, looking very strangely, we are told, as they glared out of the fog; drunk with passion of some sort, if not with brandy; and, as Sergeant Jowett writes, "shouting like madmen." It appeared afterwards that these were not the first Russians seen that morning, though it was only six o'clock. A party of unarmed Russians were seen on a hill, and believed to be — what they said they were — deserters. The officer in front incautiously advanced to receive them, and was seized, with his picket, by a stronger force concealed behind. This prevented any alarm being given, till the cries of the enemy, and the opening of the battle, roused the whole force.

How that force acted that day, history will tell. How every fragment of the army, whether roused from sleep, or called from the untasted meal, or rising from a sick bed (as Sir De Lacy Evans), or left alone to hold the ground at any cost, was instantly ready, and thoroughly to be relied on, Englishmen will never forget; — nor Frenchmen either. For eight hours the struggle lasted. For hour after hour the Russians swarmed up on all sides, as if there was really no end of them. Heavy masses of them pushed one another up the steep. Long trains of them wound up the ravines. Other masses appeared in flank, where there was no provision for meeting them. There was nothing to limit their fire; for, besides their numbers, their ammunition was inexhaustible: whereas our small force was distressed for powder and ball before the struggle was half over; and the battle was fought with stones and bayonets in various directions at once. Besides their ninety guns in the field, the Russians had the aid of their armed ships in the harbour, and the Sebastopol ordnance, while the British were weak in artillery, and had no advantage in cavalry to compensate in other ways. While in the depth of the conflict, and striving to bring up more guns, the British saw their camp going to ruin under the fire from the city and harbour, which did not hurt them, but tore the tents behind them, killed their horses, and ploughed up the ground. Against such odds did our soldiers hold out for eight hours, without food or drink or pause. More than that, they could not be commanded with the usual effect. What with the extent of the field, the character of the terrain, and the thickness of the fog, their commanders could not co-operate, or could not know that they were co-operating. It was a task of dogged resistance, varied by ingenious resources, that had to be done that day; and done mainly by the men. Hence its name of "The Soldiers' Battle." The arrival of French reinforcements under General Bosquet gave a triumphant close to a day which was then, as it had been before, trembling between victory and defeat, and which ought, by all considerations of probability, to have been lost. We remember the roar of delight with which that incident was commemorated long after in the Crystal Palace. The guardsman who was in the chair at that honorary festival put a question which electrified his comrades when he asked: — "Do you remember seeing the French coming over the hill?" They came at a moment when exhausted nature would have, — not yielded, perhaps, but sunk. They gave opportunity to our broken and mingled regiments to re-form; and then the British were ready to charge again, for the relief of the French, overpowered by numbers in their turn. Together they rolled back the Russian multitude, and broke its confidence in its own crusade. In the opinion of the Russians, the war, or the Crimean part of it at least, turned on the battle of Inkerman more than any other. Their antagonists won it, and by what force?

The Russians, we are told, had at least 50,000 men engaged. The British had 8000, and the French 6000. For hours 8000 of our soldiers resisted and drove back six times their own number, and did not yield when the head of the Russian column was in their very midst, supported by enormous pressure behind. Our soldiers withstood them, drove them back, and followed them even when they were screened behind the underwood on the slope: and yet the conquerors had not fed nor drunk that day, and scarcely a man of them was in his natural vigour. A vast proportion of the army was in hospital; hence the smallness of the force on the great day of Inkerman; and grave as was the proportion of deaths in the battle, it was so small in comparison with the mortality from disease at that time as to astonish the few who then knew the real state of the case. It was not that the wounds and deaths on the field were fewer than had been expected, but that the victims of zymotic diseases were more. The number of British killed in the battle was 462; the killed, wounded, and missing together were 2612; the amount of sick during that month of November was above thirty per cent. of the force in the Crimea, only 15,303 being available out of an army of 22,057: and of the available soldiers few were in sound health and strength. In comparison with these figures, the list of casualties after the battle of Inkerman seems almost insignificant; yet it was a heavy loss, as losses in battle are. The conclusion is that the sickness was more fearful still.

Now that we have turned to contemplate the proper calamities of warfare, we must see what became of the wounded.

When an army is fighting its way near the coast, as ours was on the Alma, the only thing to be done with the wounded is to ship them off, without delay, to the General Hospital, which, it is to be supposed, is prepared for their reception. In case of a prolonged siege, or settled encampment, there is occasion for a choice whether to send the wounded to the hospital at the base of operations, or to keep them with the army. Such cases as are too severe for expectation of recovery, or for removal without extreme risk, remain on the spot; and so do the slight cases, wherein there is hope of speedy and complete recovery. The long cases, and those which involve a retirement from the service, are the classes for which the General Hospital is supposed to be prepared.

Regimental hospitals form a special characteristic of the British service. In continental states, where large armies are concentrated within small limits, the sick are treated in General Hospitals. The British army, on the contrary, is scattered in detachments over the whole face of the globe at such distances as to render any system of General Hospitals during peace impracticable, except at those few points where a sufficient number of troops are stationed. Regimental hospitals are calculated for the service of from 800 to 1000 men, provision being made for the treatment of from twenty-five to forty at a time; that is, for a few more than the average number off duty in an assemblage of 800 to 1000 men. The regimental surgeons attend, orderlies are appointed to wait on the sick, at the rate of one to every ten patients, and a superior medical officer performs inspection at intervals. Into this hospital come all who are in any way ailing in the regiment; or at least they are under the care of their medical officers, whether actually within the hospital or not. Thus there may be in ordinary times twenty patients suffering under a dozen different diseases, of different degrees of seriousness, in the same hospital; and in the field the same may be, and probably is, the case in a dozen other hospitals within hail. It would be a waste of words to argue at length the economy in every way of an organisation, which, during war, and to some extent during peace, should supersede this fragmentary method. It is a vast saving of suffering to classify the sick according to their ailments, instead of leaving each to take his chance for the most appropriate treatment among a score of fellow-sufferers who require a different treatment. Where a wardful of patients are so far in a similar condition as to need much the same medicine and mode of nursing, warmth or coolness, food and air, they can be supplied with far more ease, and certainty, and quietness, than if each were among sufferers with wholly different wants. Medicine, attendance, diet, medical comforts, bedding, clothing, sanitary appliances, everything, in fact, which can conduce to the welfare and recovery of the sick is, or ought to be, at hand in a General Hospital. Hence the benefit of General Hospitals; and hence the absurdity of the regimental method of treating the sick, wherever a real organisation is possible. If it is so in ordinary times, what must be the state of regimental hospitals in the midst of an epidemic, or after a sanguinary battle? If five hundred want accommodation and treatment out of the means provided for fifty, what are the distracted surgeons to do? The same number of doctors could treat the larger number of patients effectually if there were suitable means and accommodation. The best thing at the moment is to send as many as possible to the General Hospital; and yet, as we have seen, being sent there has till lately been regarded in the army as nearly equivalent to a sentence of death.

Going to Scutari.—Eight thousand British, we have been told, fought at Inkerman. Thousands more were at their posts, keeping the widely extended lines; but there were also two thousand sick. When two thousand wounded were thrown on the hands of the surgeons, who were before reporting that they were overwhelmed with patients, and destitute of the means of treating them, there was clearly nothing to be done but to ship off the largest possible number to Scutari. It was a melancholy transaction,— that of embarking and disembarking soldiers at Balaclava at that time. Those who were carried on board were the fine trained troops whom we had dismissed so proudly from our shores, or who had come to the Crimea from distant quarters where they had passed stoutly through every trial of climate or service. They were our best troops,— not only costly, but unreplaceable, who were going to meet their hospital doom: whereas the reinforcements who came into the harbour as the others went out, were raw soldiers, levied in haste, half disciplined, and wholly inexperienced in hardships, and indeed in any varieties of living. During that winter one regiment, some of us may remember, lost more men than it was calculated to turn out for service on the average.

The Transport. — Fifty sick-transports carried the hospital patients to Scutari between the landing in the Crimea in September and the end of January. Some were steamers and some sailing vessels; the voyage from Balaclava being less than two days for the former, and six for the latter, on an average. Considering that the errand of the army in the Crimea was war, it seems natural that arrangements should have been made from the outset to fit up as hospitals as many sick-transports as might probably be wanted, to keep them in a cleanly and ready condition, and to provide for their being rapidly filled, and speedily despatched, after a battle. As there were sure to be cases too grave for removal, a hospital at Balaclava was obviously wanted. Yet it was an average of eight days and a half that the patients were kept on board the transports. First, they were carried over the almost impassable six miles from the camp to the harbour: and then they lay in their narrow quarters, on board dirty, close, and crowded ships, for above a week, — aware that the steamers were making, or could make, the voyage each way, while they were waiting to set sail, and might again pass them twice before they should land. There was less crowding in the latter part of the voyage, — so large a number were committed to the deep. Nearly a thousand died on that passage in the four months and a half. During the month in which the Inkerman battle was fought, 162 died in the voyage to Scutari, out of 2981 embarked. Of the desperately sick and wounded left at Balaclava, a much smaller proportion died than of the more hopeful cases at sea.

The question is simply whether the vessels were unfit for the reception of the patients, or whether the patients were in an unfit state to be put on board the vessels. As for the first, no knowledge seemed to exist of the quantity of air required for an assemblage of people who could not spend the day on deck, as passengers usually do at sea. "Ventilation" was not forgotten, so far as securing a passage of air is concerned; but the space allotted to each recumbent man was appointed without any computation of the height between decks. The surgeons were so much wanted in camp that there was a deficiency at sea. That one surgeon should be expected to attend any number above a hundred, some of whom had wounds requiring close and constant care, seems now like insanity. As to the alternative—that the patients were not fit to be passengers — it is enough to say that several were sick of choleraic disease.

Boats were ready in the harbour at Balaclava, unless a verbal message bespeaking them failed to be delivered. It was a question whether few or many of the passengers should be sent down at once. If few, they lay rocking on the sea till the whole number had arrived. If several hundreds, some lay exposed on the beach while the boats went backwards and forwards with their helpless freight. Such as died on the beach were put under ground in their red coats, as quickly as possible, in the cemetery, which was afterwards taken such good care of. When the chief medical officer was told that there was a transport, now full and ready to start, he sent on board two, three, or more surgeons, as he supposed they could be spared. He did not necessarily know the names of the vessels; it had been no part of his business to prepare the means of transport. Nor was it apparently anybody's business to see that there were mattresses and blankets enough for the men, and proper means of giving them their food. They were waited on by orderlies who were unaccustomed to the sea, and therefore disabled by sea-sickness. But these nurses themselves were invalids before they came on board, being, for the most part, taken from the invalid depôt at Balaclava. There were only four of them to every hundred patients. Several became patients, and added to the distress and confusion. Some were only sea-sick; and some were disorderly. The surgeons had no power over them beyond the threat of reporting them; and, in all these troubles, there was nothing for it but the surgeons doing everything themselves. Dreary days of confusion like this, followed by nights in which there was little rest for anybody, while the dead were stolen away from among the living, as might best be done, and let down into the deep waters — more every night; these were features of the transport service of that winter, which made it a detested service to all concerned. Towards the end of the winter, however, there was some improvement. The cases had a more hopeful aspect; the vessels and their preparation were more fit for duty; and the mortality on board diminished from ninety to nineteen per thousand.

It was a chance what the sufferers found at the other end of their voyage. Notice that they were coming might or might not have been given to the authorities at the Scutari hospitals; and they might or might not have been able to secure the speedy landing and housing of the sufferers.*

Scutari Hospitals.—In August, Lord Raglan, aware that there must soon be wounded to be cared

* There were four of these hospitals, one only of which was ever intended to receive sick. First, there was the General Hospital, a vast building erected by the Turks as a military hospital. Next, there was a large barrack, holding about ten thousand Turkish soldiers, crowded together to an inconceivable extent. Subsequently, a palace belonging to the Sultan, in a wet unhealthy position, was opened as a hospital after the two great buildings had been filled so full of sick that they could hold no more. When this too was filled, a set of miserable dens over a cavalry stable were resorted to as a shelter for the overflow. Another great cavalry barrack, with its hospital, situated at Koulali, about three miles up the Bosphorus, was fitted up as a General Hospital; and, as it was the worst, it was also the most destructive to human life of all the hospitals on the Bosphorus.

for (though as far as any one from foreseeing epidemics), gave warning about preparing Scutari hospitals for use. Three months were wasted; six weeks before the patients began to pour in, and six weeks afterwards. But it was not then known as it is now what is meant by preparing a General Hospital for use. There could be no clear idea on the subject while medical men and military officers supposed that a collection of regimental hospitals was the same thing as a General Hospital. The authorities professed to follow, as far as possible, the general rules for regimental hospitals; the employment and inspection of the medical officers had the same features, —the inspection relating to anything rather than the medical or surgical practice; and in theory, and wherever it could be achieved in practice, the grouping of the patients in regimental fashion, rather than the distribution of them under organic arrangements, was the aim. There had been no practice in the use of organised General Hospitals in time of peace; and it was no wonder that nobody thought of it, or knew how to set about it at the outset of a war.

Preparations.—Complaints were made in the hot weather of 1854, before the landing in the Crimea, of certain causes of mischief,—a catgut manufactory and other nuisances,—near the General Hospital at Scutari; and the inspecting authorities soon after declared that great improvement had been wrought, within and without, and that sanitary measures should be strictly attended to in future. The Barrack Hospital had been in a still worse state,—indescribably offensive from the stoppage of drains and the bursting of pipes, and the saturation of parts of the building with filth; and this was the edifice which was proposed to be prepared for the reception of the sick by the rooms being "well washed out, and the walls and passages white-washed." In reading the correspondence, the strangest impression is produced by the vagueness of the instructions and suggestions, in a matter of such practical importance as the care of the wounded and sick. There are directions to exercise attention, in regard to nuisances and sanitary practices; but no man tells any other man, in a business-like way, what to do. It is seldom that we get so far on firm ground as the mention of white-washing. It seems as if, through the whole series of persons, each had exhorted somebody else to observe; but that nothing came of it. There was no sanitary department organised; whatever was done was a sort of extra work of somebody, who had his own proper business to attend to; and of course there was neglect, and nobody rightfully answerable for it. Amidst such confusion, it is not very wonderful that the hospitals at Scutari were what they were found to be by the poor fellows who were carried into them after the battle of Inkerman.

The Abode.—The large buildings were sure to be

cold in winter; and inquiry was made in November as to how warmth was to be provided. There was no answer, and nothing was seen to be done during that month; but early in December it was ascertained from an engineer officer that it was to be hoped that stoves would be put up in the General Hospital (as they were already in the Barrack Hospital), by the 18th of the month (within a week of Christmas-day); but that the date could not be relied on, as the work was to be done by Turks, at the desire of the Turkish government. In the Barrack Hospital, so sufficiently warmed, the temperature was such that the medical officers would not allow the windows to be open. Yet this was the only means of ventilation in a building so abounding in stenches as to be absolutely intolerable to those who entered it from the open air. The General Hospital was better ventilated than the other,—somewhat less poisonous from the exclusion of air; but as to the quality of what the men breathed, it may be judged of by some of the facts on record.

Officers who had returned to England told of the infamous state of the sewerage in and about the Scutari hospitals; and in January 1855, the *chef* in London wrote to inquire whether the sewers had been attended to, and also the burial-ground. The answer in February was that the sewers and pipes were "a subject of consideration," and were then undergoing a course of cleaning;—then, in February, after the catastrophe was near its end, no less than 1473 soldiers having been buried from the hospitals in January! The graves were very close to the General Hospital; the ground within the Barrack Hospital square was wet, from being insufficiently drained; six dead dogs lay just under one ward window, and a dead horse "for some weeks in the aqueduct!" The floors of the Barrack Hospital were so rotten that they must be left dirty, or produce erysipelas if they were washed: and they would not dry,—those which were washed in the morning being still wet at night. Every part of the building seemed to be infested with animal matter;—the walls and ceilings gave out pestilence from this cause; and the filth, vermin, and rats, alive and dead, under the wooden divans on which the men lay, were in themselves a sufficient poison. Such was the place, as an abode, to which the wounded and sick were brought from Balaclava. Such was its condition when there had been several months' grace for getting it into order. If any due conception of a General Hospital had been entertained, there would have been, not only a removal of all existing filth, but arrangements for rendering harmless, and carrying away, all the refuse from an abode containing 2000 persons. There would have been a provision of pure water, accessible wherever it was wanted in the building, and security against all pollution of it. There would have been new floors, and a new treatment of the walls and ceilings, and new openings for ventilation, and sufficient means of warmth. Leaving out, for the moment, all considerations but of the mere housing of the patients,— which of course includes ventilation, it appears that nothing effectual was done to prevent the poisoning of thousands of our invalid soldiers by a foul atmosphere;— for want, as it seems, of a department properly charged with such precautions.

The structure of these buildings, and the defects and dilapidations may be ascribed to Turkish management. When we come to consider the accommodations for the expected inmates, we can no longer lay the blame, nor any considerable part of the blame, of mismanagement on the Turks. It was in the summer, when some of our force was going to Varna, that the Scutari hospitals were allotted to our troops; and there was a long interval for furnishing purposes between that allotment and the battle of Inkerman, which filled the hospitals to overflowing.

Registration of Patients.—Before the wounded from the camp could be landed, it was understood that they must be accounted for by a register which the chief surgeon on board the transport was expected to furnish. It too often happened that the return was not ready; and the sufferers could not be received on shore till it was completed. That was the theory. But the surgeons were, at best, cruelly perplexed to perform the services urgently required at sea, and could not spare a moment to prepare returns of names, military description, wounds, or diseases, &c., which it cost half a day to make out. In some instances the chief surgeon was down in fever; and then his assistant was under double stress. Sometimes the officer at Scutari made out, or obtained, a return at once, and sent the sufferers ashore; sometimes they were detained; and sometimes the return was omitted. Throughout the whole scene of the war there seems to have been an incessant struggle to get returns out of medical men, and on the part of each medical man to make the returns required of him, on various matters which non-medical men could have done as well or better; while the dearth of medical and surgical care was heart-breaking. We shall have occasion by and by to see what has been learned by experience of the best methods of obtaining sound statistical information, medical and other; part of the experience which has so instructed us being that of the miserable effects of occupying surgeons with making lists and tables and records of facts which there would be more reason for assigning to almost any other set of men in the whole expedition.

At the landing-place, or at the hospital-gate, the adjutant or his sergeant took the names of all who were able to speak, and applied to the officer in charge for the list of those who had died on the voyage. No register of the sick received was at that time kept at the Hospital; and the death of a patient was known only by the disappearance of his name from the orders for food, or by the list of burials kept by the adjutant. If the surgeons on board succeeded in making a return, it went into the medical office, and afforded no guidance in the wards. There the duty, again, fell on the overworked surgeons. If the Inkerman sufferers entered at night, the assistant surgeon, who was to attend perhaps a hundred of them, was required to report the particulars of every case of the hundred by nine the next morning; and in addition to those professional particulars, an account of the soldiers' names, regiment, regimental number, &c., which should have been the business of a Department of Registration. No wonder it was a common circumstance for several to die before they could give their names. While this state of things went on it was impossible to ascertain the truth about the deaths. In that very November the Hospital list reported twelve fewer deaths than were recorded in the orderly room: in December 143, and in January 125 fewer; — that is, in three months, 280 deaths were unnoticed in the Hospital report. During the preceding month and the following, October and February, the mistake was the other way; 12 deaths in October, and 253 in February being set down in excess of the orderly-room returns. But the adjutant's burial list showed both the others to be below the mark, — 280 more men having been buried than were returned as dead.

Again, the census taken in the following April proved that no less than 517 non-commissioned officers and soldiers had been buried, whose deaths were unrecorded. These were struck off the strength of the army; but there remained 28 whose names and regiments were never discovered. So painful a kind of confusion as this, in regard to the first soldiers who suffered in actual battle, was naturally put an end to with no great delay. By the end of March the disorder ceased; and in April, as I have said, a census of the Hospitals was taken, and the results compared, and brought into agreement with the returns of the Adjutant-general in the Crimea. The numbers finally reported to us are these: The General Hospital contained 800, and the Barrack Hospital 1,500 when Miss Nightingale arrived. From June 1854, to June 1856 inclusive, there were received into the General Hospitals on the Bosphorus, 43,288 sick and wounded soldiers — of whom 5,432 died. What an idea it gives us of the vast importance of hygiene in war to know that, out of this mighty host of sick, dying, and dead, fire and sword contributed only 4,161 admissions, and 395 deaths during the entire period!

Once within the gates of either hospital, what next for the sufferers?

Clothes. — Many of them were carried in almost destitute of clothing in that November weather. They had lain on deck, some of them, on a single blanket; and that single blanket, probably, was swarming with vermin, as it now covered their shoulders. A pair of ragged trousers and a forage cap might be all besides. Many had no shirt. It seems natural that among the preparations for hundreds of wounded men, proper bedding and dress for hospital-life would have been nearly the first. It was so once, the medical witnesses tell us. The hospital Purveyor used to provide stocks of sheets, shirts, flannel garments, stockings, combs, &c., which were supplied to the sick as needed. From a notion that it would be more economical for each soldier to bring his pack with him, containing two shirts, knife, fork, spoon, brushes, &c., it was long ago (since 1817) ordered that the supply of these things from hospital stores should cease. Though it was known two months before that the soldiers had thrown away, or sent to the ships, all they had hitherto carried, even, in many cases, their camp-kettles; the authorities conceived that they "had to assume that the soldier's pack would be brought with him to Scutari, and that his two shirts would be available for his use, as well as his knife, fork, spoon, &c." Such things being proved "to be not forthcoming," a requisition for 60,000 cotton shirts was sent to England in October.

The number of admissions to hospital during the three following months was just 11,000. Up to the middle of that time, the number of shirts in the knapsacks of patients was twenty-two. Those which were on their persons were often so filthy that they were at once cut off and burnt. It may therefore be said that these 11,000 patients had to be provided with shirts, within three months, and 2,000 more who were already in the Scutari wards. Considering the nature of the wounds, and the illnesses, and the bareness of those hospitals, and the difficulty about washing, a very large supply was necessary. The authorities gave out nearly 14,000, which, of course, afforded no change. Before the middle of November, however, there was some relief. Within three months from that time, Miss Nightingale issued, from her private stores, shirts to the number of 16,560. With this aid, the number was less than three shirts per man; not too much for a man in health and with facilities for washing, and far too little for helpless patients with bleeding and discharging wounds, cholera, or fever; but what could have been done without that additional supply? Some of the poor fellows from the camp must have wondered what could be done when they were laid down, in their rags or naked, on their beds at Scutari. And what were the beds?

Beds. — An abundance of sheets, fit to meet any demand, had been reported. But the poor men could not lie on those sheets, which were of a canvas so coarse as to be a real torture to the emaciated and suffering patients. They entreated to have the sheets removed, and to be left in their blankets. The blankets brought in with the men, and those in which they lay, swarmed with vermin to an extent which could not be credited without reading the testimony of witnesses; but there was no deficiency of them. In the General Hospital, the number of bedsteads was sufficient for the occupants expected; the Turks having left some of theirs. In the other hospital few of the patients had bedsteads in November; and the number of iron ones was too small throughout. By degrees, boards and trestles were supplied, till all were raised off the ground; but a great number suffered severely from the deficiency of bedsteads. We have seen something of what was under the divans on which the men lay; but there was other mischief. The floors of the corridors, where the patients lay close packed in rows, were flagged with stone or tiles; and on this floor, covered with a mat, were the men laid, on paillasses, with no relief from the cold unyielding hardness of such a bed, except in a few extreme cases, in which a hair-mattress was allowed. This happened in an eastern country, where people carry their beds about with them, and where every traveller, to say nothing of every resident, has his little mattress of cotton. Any quantity could have been got in Constantinople, at any time. The sufferers did not complain; for no one ever seems to have asked for luxury, in any form; and they perhaps considered a bed less hard than a board a luxury; but their nurses saw the fatal effect of the pain and sleeplessness thus caused, and have said that no patient ought ever again to be laid on a paillasse without a mattress. It may be unnecessary to say also, that every man should have a bedstead which admits of a constant passage of air, and preservation of cleanliness below him.

Ventilation.—But even these evils seem to grow less in our eyes when we think of the fatal mischief of want of air, which killed more of our soldiers than any other cause whatever. We know, or seem to know, far too little yet about our human need of air where we have the choice how to live in our own homes. It is no wonder that in Turkish hospitals the principles of due ventilation are not understood; and when crowding became, to all appearance, absolutely necessary, it was not to be expected that any vacant room, however small, would be refused for the reason that there were already too many for the supply of air.

It is of great importance that people should know what they mean when they talk of "overcrowding" as a cause of sickness and death; for no little confusion exists on that point. No doubt there are great evils in people being huddled together, in any place and at any time. The rear ranks of soldiers on a march are more distressed than the front rank. The men in front meet the air from head to foot, and what they meet is fresh; whereas the men in the rear are walled up by their comrades, and they march into the breath of those who are before them. Apart from the mechanical pressure in a dense crowd, in the open air, we are sensible of oppression and difficulty of breathing. Our proper quantity of fresh air is interfered with by the number of people about us, and we are consuming some of theirs, whatever quantity there may be overhead. We are told that when once we have sixteen feet overhead, any further amount is of little consequence; but that we suffer more or less unless we have a sufficiency around us. Thus far we may speak of crowding as an evil; but we are too apt to consider the crowding as the fatal mischief in itself, which it is not. The fatal mischief is the insufficiency of air fit for breathing. The practical effect of the confusion is, that it leads the attention away from the main question,—how to supply the largest quantity, and most constant renewal of the air to the people contained within a certain area. In short, we think too little of the height and ventilation of apartments, in comparison with the area of the floor. What we call the "Black Hole" at Calcutta, was not an airless dungeon: it was an apartment in which two persons could have lived very pleasantly, with the window open: but the height did not allow a supply for more. If a hurricane had that night carried off the roof, the prisoners would have been found alive in the morning, to a man. They would have been weary for want of room for many to lie down. They would have been more or less heated and oppressed: but no one need have been suffocated, or could have been poisoned with foul air. A crowd in a tea-garden to see a balloon go up, or a throng in the park to see the Queen go to open parliament, does not complain of being stifled, whatever other inconvenience it may suffer. It would be wiser, if we could learn to do it, to speak of the cubic space that people live in, than the length and breadth of the floor, in considering which we are too apt to forget the height of the ceiling, and the position of the windows. It is a great evil, certainly, that in any cottage or lodging-house, a dozen people should live day and night in a room of ten feet square; but they might do it in a Malay country without injury to health,—on a platform on posts, that is, with a thatch roof overhead, and no walls, or a mere open lattice. They might do it in certain ancient hypæthral temples,—temples with massive walls and no roof. When we have thoroughly surmounted this confusion about "overcrowding," and have learned that the thing essentially wanted is a certain number of cubic feet of fresh air per minute for each individual, we shall understand precisely what the mischief of "overcrowding" is, viz., a secondary evil which may be greatly mitigated by a continual influx of fresh air, unless the crowding be so great as to render this impossible. When we have practically cleared our minds of all confusion, that is, when we act on our common sense, we shall hear no more of fevers, cholera, or any kind of hospital plague. Meantime, a tragedy like that of Scutari will now and then occur, with the additional horror (unless the clear heads interfere in time) that any such calamity is henceforth a crime, and that what we have hitherto called mortality, becomes murder from this time forward.

What cubic space ought each individual to have, in order that his life may be duly sustained by the air he breathes? Considering the hospital case alone, what is the proper allowance there? Dr. Christison's account of the matter is regarded as authority by the best informed persons. Supposing the height from the men's pillows to the ceiling to be fourteen feet (and it ought not to be less) their beads should be at least nine feet apart, and ten feet from the middle of the ward. The space assigned as essential is 1300 cubic feet per man; but this supposes an unremitting change of air, to the extent of at least 4000 cubic feet per man per hour. In the London civil hospitals, the cubic space allowed is from 1300 to 2000 feet. In our naval hospitals it is from 1200 to 1500. How is it with our soldiers? In our military hospitals the allowance is from 500 to 700 feet; and in our barracks it has hitherto been from 300 to 500, — that miserable supply being lessened by the folly of the sufferers themselves, who are ignorantly apt to close every opening through which the smallest relief could be obtained.

Thus starved of the vital principle of the atmosphere, and poisoned with the refuse part, our soldiers might well die as they did. No description of "over-crowding," as if the mischief lay in the mere huddling together, could give any idea of the murderous process by which so many thousands were sent to their graves.

How was it with the wounded from Inkerman?

The space allowed by regulation is two feet between each bed in hospital. Supposing the best possible sanitary condition of the building, this space is admitted on all hands to be not more than half what it ought to be. At best, therefore, the patients could not be expected to do well. But the sanitary condition was fearfully bad; and thus it was certain that the patients must do badly. What was to be anticipated when the insufficient space was again divided, and twice as many were admitted as had been reckoned on? What but a fearful mortality could ensue? "The paillasses were laid on the floor as close as they could lie," the Evidence tells us. The corridors, by which fresh air should have been supplied, were turned into wards. They were so nearly filled by two rows of beds that two persons abreast could scarcely pass between foot and foot. That was in the Barrack Hospital, which contained for six weeks 2000 patients in the space allotted to 1220; and for another six weeks 2200 in the space allotted to 1600. The effect was of one hospital being thrust into another,— the clear spaces intended for air being occupied by the sick. When the doors were open they did not, as they ought, admit fresh air to the wards, but caused the corrupt atmosphere of wards and corridors to mingle. In the General Hospital, there was one row of beds in the corridors, and the allowance of space to each man was five feet. This was not so bad a state of things as that of the Barrack Hospital; but the men would have had a better chance in the open fields,— wintry as the season was.

The constant change of the air is more important than even the quantity at each moment. It is enough to say that in the Barrack Hospital there were no openings to the outer air,— no means of letting out the mass of foul air that gathered under the lofty ceilings. There were no open windows, no open fire-places, nor any draught up the staircases; nor was anything done for many weeks; when, at last, portions of the windows were taken out, and filled in with perforated zinc plates; and holes in the roof converted the staircases into ventilating shafts. In the General Hospital there were larger windows and more of them, so that a sufficiency of air was finally secured. Early in the winter of 1854-5, however, the patients were lying packed together in wards and corridors, where the stench was intolerable to any one coming in from the open air; and the sickness and diarrhœa, hospital gangrene among the wounded, and cholera which made an indiscriminate sweep, rapidly filled the burial-ground. Even these pestilences did not thin the hospitals; for more and more were brought from the Crimea, both wounded and sick. On the 17th of December newly-repaired wards were opened, just in time to admit a rush of patients, amounting to 4000 in seventeen days; yet the next six weeks were the period when 2200 occupied the space intended for 1600.

Something must be said about cleanliness, but it shall be as little as possible.

Cleanliness.—In a properly organised General Hospital, cleanliness is as much a matter of certainty as the giving of food. Experience shows that this part of the management should be conducted by women; and certainly the medical officers ought not to be troubled with the details of it. It is a matter of research what are the best substances of which the walls, floors, ceilings, and furniture of hospitals should be composed, with a view to cleanliness and dryness. These points ascertained, nothing should be left to chance. The proper persons should be charged with the work of removing every sort of dirt; and the times and methods of doing it should be enforced by the strictest rules. The scrubbing, sweeping, rubbing, and dusting will be provided for as in a private abode, only with more careful steadiness. As to the other causes of offence, always accruing where there are wounds, sores, and intestinal disease of all kinds, instant removal is the only rule. Even then there remains the large subject of the washing for such a throng of sick people. It would be more painful than profitable to detail the condition in which the Scutari patients lay before it was possible to institute those reforms which made all clean and comfortable at last. Suffice it that the persons of the men, and even their wounds, swarmed with vermin; that they lay, in too many instances, in indescribable filth. The clothes and bedding were put out to be washed by contract. When the quantity done was nearly sufficient, the quality of the washing was often bad, — both blankets and shirts being brought back with vermin in them, and by no means cleansed from the worst dirt they contained. The authorities did not in fact understand the necessity of boiling, to get out animal matter entirely, and no means of boiling were provided. In the other case, the Barrack Hospital, the quantity done was miserably insufficient; — the clean shirts for the patients being at times less than one per fortnight each. The poor fellows dreaded being obliged to wear other men's shirts under these circumstances; it was naturally difficult to give each man his own; and it was no uncommon thing to find four or five dirty shirts concealed in the bed of a patient who was unwilling to send them to the wash, lest he should never see them again. An effort was early made to give assistance to the Barrack Hospital; and Miss Nightingale's washing establishment supplied 2000 clean (really clean) shirts per month. We remember the drying-closet sent to Scutari by Miss Coutts, with an engineer to set it up, and see it well at work: but that was in June, 1855. The washing establishment, with its machines for boiling, wringing, and drying, came into operation on the 1st of May. Five months before, the poor fellows from Inkerman were lying, too probably, without either shirts or sheets, and in a state which it would be needlessly painful to describe. The topic would have been omitted altogether but for the credit due to the contrast presented a year later, as one of the consequences of a rational hospital organisation. The time came when every patient was lying between clean sheets and blankets, with a sufficiency of wholesome clothing, with means of ablution, and an abundance of fresh air, and freedom from bad smells; — in short, with every fair chance of recovery; but that was when nearly all the wounded from Inkerman were in their graves, or gone home invalided.

It was not from any personal disinclination for cleanliness that the patients lay in such a state. In camp, we know, they did not take off their clothes for weeks together; and their condition was bad accordingly: but they naturally supposed that they could be clean in hospital; and they eagerly desired it. But, unhappily, according to the practice of Regimental hospitals, the authorities of General Hospitals think themselves entitled to assume that each man, as well as each doctor, would bring his own soap and towels; and no preparation was made to help them to the means of washing their faces, in case of their coming in unprovided. In Regimental hospitals, there is usually in each ward one basin and one jack-towel, not necessarily transferred to a General Hospital in war. The number of towels washed for the Barrack Hospital during the three months following the 1st of November, for from 2000 to 2400 patients, was 132. At the end of that time, when there were above 2000 patients in hospital, the return of purveyor's stores shows what the provision for personal cleanliness was: viz.; 14 baths, no basins, and 194 towels. At the General Hospital the stock was increased by 200 Turkish towels, bought by Miss Nightingale at Constantinople, immediately after her arrival, subsequently increased by her from private funds on the requisition of the medical officers, to an additional supply of 5826 towels, and 624 zinc basins, besides soap, baths, brushes, combs, and scissors. Scarcely a man was known to bring one of the articles supposed to be in his kit: the Purveyor considered himself debarred from furnishing them, lest he should be supplying duplicates; and thus were the men sacrificed to the theory of a Regimental hospital when carried to a General one. In a Regimental hospital, the patient brings in his kit from his quarters, just at hand. In the General Hospital, he is brought from a distance, under circumstances unfavourable to his carrying a wardrobe : and at Scutari the consequences were seen. For the most essential means of cleanliness, the patients had to wait till they were supplied from private funds. Though the practice of personal cleanliness is an affair between the soldier and his medical officer, as we have already seen, the supply of the means is a proper head of General Hospital organisation,—no less pertinent and necessary than the provision of means for eating and sleeping, and being nursed.

As for the appliances for these wants,—what were they in November, 1854?

Implements and Utensils.—Among many forlorn pictures, perhaps the most terrible is that of a Regimental hospital tent full of cholera patients in the night, in total darkness: more and more being attacked; new cases coming in; and all in total darkness! No wonder we hear of the regimental surgeons being "horror-struck" on finding there was not a candle to be had. Almost everything in these Field Hospitals most needed was deficient. In the General Hospitals, among the articles supplied from the same private funds, on the requisition of the medical officers, there were 168 lanterns, candle-lamps, and lamps; hundreds of yards of india-rubber sheeting; bed-furniture of all kinds,—air-beds, pillows, utensils, dressing-gowns, &c., a vast supply: tin plates 2086; 208 tin pails for soup; drinking-cups 5477; spoons 2630; and so on. During the time when not a spoon, or knife and fork, or towel, or brush, was to be got for the men, hundreds of knapsacks were heaped up in the Pack-store at Scutari, unopened and unsorted. They were examined and disposed of in April, 1855, when thousands of the men had departed, dead or alive. As it was "assumed" that every man possessed the utensils for eating and drinking, and had the use of them in hospital, few or none were provided; and the benevolent people at Scutari went about, hunting up spoons, plates and basins, towels, combs and scissors, when there was a heap of stray knapsacks untouched in a store-room. The Purveyor's report shows a stock of 233 spoons, 194 towels, 674 knives and forks; and so on, in proportion, at a time when 4000 patients were sent in in seventeen days.

Food.—We are furnished with details as to the serving of the food, by which we perceive only too plainly how small a chance the patients had of withstanding hospital epidemics. In the Barrack Hospital there were two kitchens, one of which was useless for want of copper boilers, though copper boilers are in use in every house in Constantinople, and must therefore be obtainable. The other was fitted up with thirteen boilers, containing about fifty-six gallons each. These might supply food enough for the ordinary number of persons in hospital, in an ordinary way; but there was no provision for affording the diet of the sick;—special nourishment at all hours to the large proportion of patients that needed it. The process of feeding the whole number was, in the first instance, so hopelessly awkward, that how it could ever have been endured for two days together is a wonder.

The wounded comrades from the plateau were visited each morning by the surgeon, who gave his directions for the food and medical comforts which he considered advisable for each, not on that, but the following day; and the memoranda were shown to the Surgeon of the Division, who looked them over, and returned the list to the person in charge of the ward,—the Wardmaster. Meantime, the Orderlies, who were the acting nurses, were setting about getting the breakfasts ordered the morning before. Each orderly acted for a mess, consisting of about twenty-five men; and the whole company of orderlies presented themselves at half-past six at the Purveyor's store, where the steward supplied to each the quantity of bread ordered for his mess. This is the time chosen for the steward to set down in the diet-book the meals ordered for the rest of the day;—the full meals, the half meals, the slop and milk diets ordered; and the only reason given for this interruption of the business of serving out the bread was that the diet-book would be wanted after breakfast, for the marking of the diets for the next day. An hour and a half was thus used up for a business which dexterous hands could get through in a few minutes. The bread was given out in loaves, and not in portions; and the same messengers had often to go to the kitchen, to get the tea. It was three hours before the meal was eaten. When it was done, the orderlies again appeared before the steward, who was engaged for three hours more in serving out the meat, salt, and bread for dinner. The meat was weighed for each mess, and delivered in bulk to the orderly, who carried it to the kitchen to be cooked. He tied up his portion, and put a skewer into it, marked with a tally, that he might know it again; and it was often half-past one o'clock before the orderlies could get their portions admitted into the boiler. Some of the patients must be half-starved, or much of the meat half raw. While the meat was boiling, the orderlies awaited the surgeon's having done with the book, and then hastened to the store, to get the porter which was ordered, and the chickens, arrow-root, wine, lemons, brandy, sago, eggs, and other extra articles. What to do with these was the difficulty; for there was seldom room for any such cookery in the kitchen. The orderlies used to cook these messes themselves, — or try to do it, — at the ward stoves, or in their own tin canteens, or in any shed in the barrack-square, or wherever they could find a fire and anything to put upon it. Before these were ready, the general dinner was cooked; and the orderly went to the kitchen for it, bringing the whole quantity for the mess on a wooden tray into the ward, and cutting it up on the floor, or—on his bed,—into five-and-twenty pieces, with a share of bone to each. By this time it was cold, of course; and if soup formed any part of the meal, it was too unpleasant in its aspect to be swallowed by weak and disordered patients. The deficiency of plates, knives, and spoons, increased the delay and difficulty. When the meal was finished, the extra-diets had to be served. The weakest patients had to wait longest for their food; and when it came, they must eat at once all that was ordered for the day, or leave it:—they could not be served twice. After all this, the orderly had to cook and eat his own dinner, and then see about the tea for his mess. How the sufferers must have needed patience under such management! Without being at all like the young men in the colony of Batavia, who, if kept waiting for half-an-hour, are seen crying like babies for their tea, the strong man at home finds he has need of *some* patience if kept hungry for two or three hours; but, in the case of the sick, waiting for food means fainting, sinking, fever, sleeplessness, —even death. Yet the dinner which should have been served at twelve or one o'clock, was sometimes not even put into the boiler till half-past one. Too often, when it came at last, it was a cruel disappointment to the sinking sufferer, who felt as if his life depended on a few mouthfuls of warm nourishment. The meat red,—the fat cold,—the arrow-root thin and cloudy, or like cold glue;—these were the spectacles too often presented to loathing patients. Yet there might have been a hot-water table in the kitchen, on which to cut the meat into portions. There might have been an oven in the ward, in which to heat the plates. There ought to have been boilers and stoves enough to ensure every patient being served punctually. There might have been a table in the ward, properly spread for such patients as could sit up, and eat their dinner in a decent and comfortable way,—with a superintending officer to see that all were duly served. Some medical officers generously undertook this task, when there came to be a dinner table,—feeling, no doubt, the importance, in a professional view, of their patients being nourished, instead of disgusted by their food. What a change it was when Miss Nightingale and the nurses appeared, with hands full of good things at the right time!

A kitchen was established for the cooking of these extras. Miss Nightingale bought boat-loads of fuel, as it was wanted, and pails, basins, dishes, bowls, trays, hot-water tins to keep the meals warm, and whatever was wanted for the conveyance of the food to the very lips, even thirty-three "sick-feeders" being in the list of comforts provided. The arrow-root was twice as thick as before, from half the quantity; the beef-tea was hot and savoury; the drinks were administered when the tongue was parched, and the cordials when the strength was sinking. Spoonfuls of nourishment might, and did, enable many to survive the night who were just fainting to death: and the mere punctuality was no doubt the saving of many. It may be hoped that the lesson has been learned. Scientific men have turned their attention full upon the subject of hospital diet; and it is found that the economy to the public is as striking as the benefit to the patients, when the system is arranged under the advantage of our new knowledge, and of a very attainable degree of skill. If the nurses at Scutari saved two ounces of rice on every four puddings, and made thick arrow-root from half the quantity taken to make thin, simply by seeing that the water boiled properly, we may understand how further knowledge may improve the economy and the comfort to an extent not yet discerned. One single proposal is very striking as an illustration; — to vary the hospital diet to such an extent (say to ten or twelve different dinners) as not only to gratify and improve the appetite of the patients generally, but to render extra diets almost unnecessary, and thus diminish one source of expense. If, instead of the eternal boiled meat, there is in turn soup, puddings of various kinds, fish, poultry, and vegetables, all cases may be met, except the few in which slops, cordials, and a small number of special articles are required. The whole thing is got hold of by the right handle, we may hope; and nothing like the wretched feeding of the sick at Scutari need be ever witnessed again.

Mismanagement about Supply.—"How did it happen?" is the natural and necessary question. Several reasons and excuses were assigned. It was believed, till too late, that everything that could possibly be wanted was in store at Scutari. Large quantities of stores which were at Varna were ordered to be brought to Scutari so early as September, and were supposed to have arrived accordingly; whereas in November there was no sign of them, and want of transport was the cause alleged for the disappointment. It seems hard that the sick should have perished at Varna for want of comforts, and that when the sick at Scutari were perishing, some months later, it should be for want of comforts which were lying at Varna. Again, there was some misunderstanding with our ambassador at Constantinople, who was requested by the government at home to supply whatever was wanted, but was misled as to what really was wanted. Between strange scruples about asking him, and mistakes as to the deficiencies, and some want of skill at Constantinople in procuring the articles needed, there was fatal privation, till private zeal and charity intervened, and began to restore comfort and revive hope. It will not be forgotten, that in November vast stores were lost by the foundering of the Prince off Balaclava; nor that great efforts were made in England, on that loss becoming known, to supply deficiencies by private collections, as well as by official exertions. It may be, even yet, less understood that there were, taking one place with another, abundant stores, which the Supply Commissioners discovered, actually hidden away from the eyes of the very persons who should have dispensed them, besides means of obtaining fresh provisions, which required only good management to procure in any quantity. All such answers turn upon what people call accidents, as the loss of the Prince, the misunderstandings with the ambassador, the difficulty of getting goods from Varna; and some sanguine people have said that such accidents are not likely to happen again. It is needless to make any further comment, after all that has been said before, than that such accidents would have been impossible, (generally speaking) if a special department had been charged with the business of bringing the supplies and the soldiers together; and if all the official persons on the spot had been so organised as that each department — the doctors, and the military officers, the purveyors, stewards, orderlies, and hangers-on — knew precisely what it had to do, and was employed according to its capacity. The absence of such organisation turns everything into accident. The perfection of such organisation would practically exclude accident from the case, by neutralising its bad consequences.

False System.—As to the most common, or most obvious, of the evils we have been reviewing,— the bad supply of food, medicine, and comforts to each patient,—it is completely explained by the operation of the system of requisitions. Throughout the first year of the war, we find that wherever we turn there were articles of necessity or comfort wanted, which were believed to be in store, or which might possibly be in store, but which could not be got at, because some form or other stood in the way. Or, the necessary supplies were ordered, and never obtained; or declared to have been given out, and never received. There was no plain, direct way for the medical men to declare what their patients wanted, with the certainty that the things would be immediately supplied. That such a method is impossible cannot be reasonably alleged, because, in the first place, private management did effectually supply the needs of the sick at Scutari; and in the next place, the system of supply was brought to great perfection in the Crimea before the close of the war; and thirdly, it has been found possible in India, where the task is far more difficult, to provide every man in the army, whether on the march or in camp, with whatever he needs, in the way of food, clothing, shelter, and transport, as the want arose. In a General Hospital, stationed near a large city, and on the margin of the sea, there ought never to have been a deficiency of a single meal, or delay in the administration of any medicine. How the system of requisitions worked so badly,—how the army, sick and well, was so ill-provided in the neighbourhood of plenty,—we may perhaps best learn by looking at the whole method of managing a Scutari, or any other General Medical Hospital.

The object of the institution may as well be agreed upon, in the first instance. Is it not to save the lives of the sick and wounded, and restore them as quickly as possible to active life? If so, any notion of saving money, as the first principle of the case, must be, not only morally wrong, but an economical mistake. Any cumbrous machinery for checking official action, with a view to saving money, must be a loss of time, and an impediment to the cure of the sick soldiers; and, it must be understood, a sick soldier is the most expensive article that the public purse has to support. It is painful to write what may have the appearance of levity or hardness; but, while the plea of money-saving is urged in defence of proceedings which prolong the sufferings of patients, the right line of argument must be that which shows the expensiveness of sick soldiers. If asked the question plainly, whether the soldiers were or were not to be cured as quickly as possible, nobody would dream of saying anything but "yes;" and we may, therefore, proceed on the supposition that such is the common aim and desire; though the actual arrangements look like something very different.

Nine Hospital Departments.—There were, at the time of the last war, nine departments in the general hospitals. The Medical Department comes first; and next the Commissariat, which is bound to carry the stores, to keep them, and to be the banker. These are the duties of the Commissariat, whether on a great scale, as in regard to the whole army, or on the smaller scale of any portion of it. The Purveyor's department is the third. It was the Purveyor's duty to receive the stores supplied by the Commissariat, and to give them out, with such other supplies as might be ordered by warrants of the War Department, and the requisitions of medical officers. The kitchen was included in the Purveyor's departm nt; and the washing, and the care of the soldier's kit, arms, accoutrements, and money.

A new class of duties appears with the fourth department, the Engineer's. His business was, not to act as a sanitary officer, but to look after the fittings, drainage, and repairs of the hospital, under the orders of military and medical authorities on the establishment. The fifth department was the Adjutant-General's,—difficult to describe, but eminently useful. He supplied parties of soldiers for all purposes, — the landing of the sick, the cleaning of the yards, and the burial of the dead; and on him depended the preservation of the military discipline. The sixth was the Quartermaster-General's, whose function is easily understood; viz., the providing of quarters for everybody,—from the highest officer to the humblest soldier's wife, within and without the hospital. He had to transport the sick, find store-room, and keep his own stores.

Then we come round again to an office of supply,—the Contractor's, with whom the Commissariat made contracts for provisions and fuel. There seems to be no little confusion between these two departments and the Purveyor's.

There remain the Pay-master's function, and the Commandant's, the titles of which seem to speak for themselves. But it would scarcely occur to any imagination what is included in the first. The Pay-master has to keep the accounts of the soldiers in hospital; that is, to receive from the Purveyor the account of the stoppages of every man in the place every day. Now, there are actually thirteen kinds of stoppage in the army; viz., two on board ship; two in the field; two for sick and wounded in the field; three for sick in hospital; one for troops at home; and three for troops serving abroad. The endless work and confusion caused by these varieties must be a greater evil than any conceivable advantage can compensate. The soldiers are never satisfied; for their accounts can never get settled to everybody's clear conviction. Many soldiers are taken from their proper business to keep the accounts. It cannot be invariably ascertained what every man's stoppage should be every day; and the soldier, the regimental Pay-master, the Purveyor, and the Commissariat are all troubled by the impossibility of getting their accounts closed. It would cost no more to the country to have a uniform stoppage; and it would be a great weight off many minds. The mere mass of accounts in a hospital containing several thousand patients, where the daily stoppage of each man had to be ascertained, calculated, and deducted from his pay may be conceived with difficulty. Yet this was a portion of the Pay-master's duty. If he could have reckoned the soldiers all round at three-pence halfpenny or four-pence halfpenny a head, what an indescribable relief it would have been to all parties concerned!

The Commandant had to command everybody and everything; not only all the soldiers in depôt and in hospital, and all military proceedings in connection with both, but the medical officers, the civil officers, and the whole mass of camp followers and labourers. As a military officer cannot be qualified to control medical management, or the business of the Purveyor's department, one of two things must happen,—either the Commandant will meddle with what he does not understand (conscientiously, no doubt), or he will leave the medical and civil officers to do their work in their own way,—without any control at all, and therefore without any unity of system. The latter method for the most part prevailed at Scutari; and, indeed, the Commandant had no official authority to obtain from the Commissariat any money or credit beyond his current official expenses. When we look a little into the mutual operation of all these offices, we shall see that the getting through the crisis at all, and the restoration of the army, were owing, not to any existing organisation, but to a setting aside of all rules, and an expenditure without limit. Money was poured out like water, and rules and regulations gave way like sand.

Medical Department. — The first body of officers that one thinks of in a hospital are the medical men. Their duty, as explained by the Director-general, was to take care that every patient was supplied with whatever he needed, without regard to expense; and, again, to take care that the men were not supplied with anything which was not needed, and which must, therefore, be hurtful. When these powers and duties were confided to the doctors, and when it was reported from Scutari that every article of necessity and comfort was stored up there in abundance, the authorities at home had no other idea than that all would go well, and expected a favourable account of the recovery of the patients. As matters turned out, what could the doctors do?

The depôt was on the spot,—in the Barrack Hospital; and the crowding of the soldiers and their wives, and the hangers-on of a depôt, caused fever, and aggravated all the mischief in the wards. If there had been a Governor of the hospital, instead of a Commandant of hospital and depôt at once, this evil would have been absent. What the crowding of the corridors was we have seen. The medical men could do nothing in regard to this fatal evil. Their field of labour was not prepared by any sanitary officials; and foul gases were whiffed into the buildings from the sewers by changes of wind, in addition to the constant grievance of insufficient ventilation. One would think that these disabilities were enough; but there were others, no less fatal. It was fearful enough that after performing secondary amputation on forty men, they saw thirty-nine of them die; and that eighty cases of hospital-gangrene were recorded in November alone,—very many more being unrecorded; but, in addition to these miseries, resulting from bad air and previous depression, there was a heart-breaking inability to get their patients fed and nursed. Their commission, received from the Director-general at home, must have looked like a cruel irony.

It had never been clearly settled what was the duty of the medical officers; so that there was endless confusion about what each should be doing. The surgeon might be seen receiving, examining, and dispensing food and wine, when he was sorely needed by the bedside of the wounded. It was calamitous; but not so much so as the other alternative of leaving his patients without food. He might be seen early in the morning directing the sweeping and cleaning of the wards; or in the kitchen, boiling starch for bandages, because his orderlies did not know how to do it; or spending hours with pen in hand, over accounts or returns, or records which could have been better kept by another man, while there was an actual deficiency of surgeons, and an epidemic in the place. As one consequence, the assistant surgeon, whose proper business it was to dress wounds and sores, and make up medicines, and fill up the diet-rolls for his superior, was charged with the duties of that superior, before it could be ascertained whether he was qualified. It is literally true that while medical officers of proved skill were in unequalled demand in the wards, some were examining corks and tasting wines, and others were at the desk for hours of the day,—their dressers and assistants having each the sole charge of sixty or a hundred grave cases. When it is added that there were several surgeries, supplied each with its own apparatus and dispenser, instead of a great organised dispensary where, by division of labour, the business might have been done rapidly, effectively, and economically in comparison, we see how far the patients and their doctors were from having had any justice in the Scutari hospitals, when the wounded from the Alma and Inkerman entered then.

System of Requisitions. — This brings us to the point of the system of requisitions. It has been said that, under that system, we arrive at an incalculable amount of papers, and at little else.

Who provided the supplies? who issued them? and on what authority?

The Commissariat and the Purveyor.—The Commissariat was charged with supplying the meat, bread, and fuel. The Purveyor was to receive the supplies, and to give them out on requisition. The Commissariat conveyed everything, and, among other articles, the medicines and implements and utensils needed. If they were in store when demanded, the Purveyor was bound to supply them; if not, he had nothing to do but to say so. As there was a steward to do the actual business of weighing out the food, it seems difficult to understand what the Purveyor was for: and indeed his office seems not to have been clearly defined. Sometimes he was told that a batch of patients was expected, and that there must be beds and food ready for them; but again, he might know nothing about them till the list of their wants was handed to him next morning. Sometimes a Purveyor would furnish no fowls or eggs for weeks together, though they were ordered, and were obtainable in the market; and in one case (speaking of eastern hospitals generally) the implements for whitewashing the wards were refused, repeatedly, though they were actually in store. Under such uncertainty, the only certain thing was that the requirements of the sick could not be fulfilled. The doctors wrote down what they desired each patient to have. The requisition was either fulfilled, or the material was supplied in part, or not at all. But the requisition remained on record, often without any notice of its not being fulfilled: and this of course introduced utter confusion into the accounts, and opened the door to waste and loss of every kind. The materials required were set down as supplied, as a matter of course: and if they were supplied at a subsequent period, they were set down again. Between the Commissariat and the Purveyor's department, there were stores which were not known to exist (like the rice and lime-juice in the Crimea, hidden out of sight when the men were sinking in dysentery, scurvy, and cholera); and, on the other hand, articles of prime necessity were absent which everybody else could get in the market. Doctors, nurses, and friends bought fowls, eggs, milk, &c. when the Purveyor failed to supply them; and there were instances when a person of courageous benevolence took the responsibility of laying hands on articles in store, whether beds or food, without going through forms which would have caused fatal delay.

The same processes were gone through about medicines. The surgery was attended at certain hours by a dispenser. In the intervals, it might be locked or open, and the dispenser might or might not be there. The surgeons might have entered, and made up a batch of medicines. Thieves might have been there, and have stolen cordials or drugs for sale. Orderlies might have been there with hasty requisitions for medicines urgently wanted. All these things were left to chance; and what chance was there that the doctors' requisitions would be responded to with any accuracy, on the one hand, or the dispensary accounts correctly kept, on the other? The only excuse for so much writing,—such requisitions, replies, records, &c. is the check thereby imposed on waste and dishonesty; but, under the so-called system, we have hitherto had to suffer all the waste of time, thought, temper, and welfare of the soldier, involved in the plan of requisitions, without obtaining thereby any security about the stores, or any result but a pure misleading of everybody's mind. It is enough to say that a large amount of things are set down as served to Miss Nightingale which she never received; while 200 Turkish towels purchased by her for the Barrack Hospital were, by mistake, carried to the General Hospital, and set down among the public stores furnished there. Incidents like these, happening daily, and, sooner or later, to every person concerned in drawing stores, show that the system of requisitions was not made to work.

The system proceeds on the supposition that nothing is issued but on a written demand; that the written demand remains as a voucher for the receipt of the articles set down in it; and that such requisitions as are not complied with are filed by themselves. If there could be any security provided for these rules being observed, the method would be very cumbrous in comparison with the ordinary practice of giving receipts for articles actually furnished. But no such security existed amidst the hurry and pressure of circumstances, in the Crimea and at Scutari: and the system broke down in every way. It was seldom possible to supply all the articles in a list, and there was not time to specify, on all occasions, what was supplied and what omitted; and there seems to have been no certainty in the filing of the requisitions which were not fulfilled, or of any note being made, to secure a supply when the articles arrived. Many articles were obtained by violation of rules, in cases of pressing need, in the absence, or under the refusal, of the proper order; many which were ordered were never obtained; there was nothing like correspondence between the written demands and the supplies actually furnished; private gifts were occasionally included among public stores, and the medical officers and nurses were declared to have received stores which were never supplied. We are told in the Evidence that if a surgeon asked for anything, — say bedsteads,—and was told there were none, his patients had to do without,—to lie on the floor; and, as everybody knew the reason, nobody asked for bedsteads, aware that it would be in vain. In one case, 289 bedsteads were deficient in one hospital. But meantime boards and trestles had arrived, and were even noted down in the Purveyor's list; but the doctors were not aware of it, and their patients continued to lie on the floor while the boards and trestles incumbered the Purveyor's over-crowded storehouse. When we have done with the complications of hospital management, as it has been, we shall see how simple are the means recommended to Government for the better issue of stores in future.

Thus we see how the medical officers have been driven to act as purveyors, accountants, ward-masters, cooks, dispensers and nurses, while they were actually too few for their proper business. When they were needed at the bed-side, or the operating table, they were absent on affairs in which their professional qualifications were lost. It is hard to say whether the trial was most severe to them, or to the sick and wounded; but rules, and the absence of rules, were alike against them. By the rules of their service, they must fill up returns, superintend the washing, examine stores, and keep accounts which could have been done better by other men; and when all was at sixes and sevens, their humanity impelled them to do whatever was most wanted; whether making a poultice, or getting the ward cleaned. There was something more required of them; quite unreasonably, and of course ineffectually. They were made the statisticians of the health and sickness of the army, and especially of the part of it which was in the hospitals. Our present business is with the latter.

Hospital Statistics. — There seems to be as much reason for the appointment of a statistical as a sanitary member of the Council, which should advise the Director-General on the health of the army. It is of high importance to know all the facts of the condition of young men who are either accepted or rejected as recruits. It is of high importance to know every fact that can be gathered about the numbers of soldiers who suffer under various diseases, in various circumstances, so that we may learn to avoid the causes of each, and to ascertain the conditions of the best health possible to an army. It is of high importance to register the sick and the wounded who enter the hospitals, and who leave it, dead, invalided, or in restored health. It is of high importance that the mortality of the army, and of all its scattered portions, should be clearly ascertained and recorded, for comparison with the mortality of other bodies or classes of men. There is reason to suppose that an efficient Statistical Department attached to the army would save more lives, and intercept more sickness, than any Medical Department ever yet established by the War-office. To charge the Medical Department with all that business, in addition to its own, would be as absurd as to require it to undertake the entire sanitary department with out increase of numbers.

It may be objected that medical officers alone are qualified, because an accurate knowledge of diseases is necessary to any sound classification of maladies, and of the facts relating to them. No doubt, the pathological reporting must be done by medical men. They must note down the more important facts of their own practice; having the discretion left them (a discretion due to their position) what special cases to record, and what to report merely as a fact. That they should do this much reporting is necessary to the advancement of medical and surgical science and practice. Such knowledge is sadly needed, for the sake of an improved classification and nomenclature of diseases; in short, for a fuller knowledge of the natural history of diseases. But all reports of this kind, and of several other kinds, are but the materials for the statistical records which it should be the business of a separate department to prepare, and to utilise for scientific purposes. But there were actual embarrassments thrown in the way of the medical men by the hospital rules at Scutari, which added to the burden of their impossible task. In the hurry and confusion of the arrival of large numbers of sick or wounded, the surgeons had to declare the nature of each man's disease or wound, for description on his ticket. We have seen how an assistant-surgeon may have to register the names, and supply the cases of a hundred new patients between night and morning. If the first impression of the case gives way before further observation, or if the aspect of it changes, the description and the ticket have to be changed, and the patient is liable to be reckoned as two men. Here is room for mistake in the register at once, to say nothing now of the errors caused in the description and estimate of diseases. If individuals were occasionally reckoned twice over, living or dying, the return of deaths was, on the whole, very far below the actual number; which indicates a most serious defect in the estimate of mortality, at another stage of the record. No one who has read the Evidence can wonder at this. The utter absence of any principle of guidance in reckoning the proportions of sick and dead to the healthy; the variations between the very terms of comparison, where the proportions of sick or dead in the week, or the month, or the year, were confounded; and the fallacious use of so-called averages where no average was obtainable, all point to the necessity of establishing a department, whose business it should be to conduct all such computations with the same accuracy that is required in a merchant's office, or at the Board of Trade. If such a department had existed during the long peace, we should not have lost the valuable records of the Walcheren expedition and the Peninsular war. They were destroyed, because they were too bulky for the convenience of the Director-General; and all that valuable experience remains a mere tradition. Unless an effort is speedily made to secure the organisation of a Statistical Department, apart from the strictly medical service, the records of the state of the army may, at any time, be as defective as they were in the Crimea and at Scutari.

By the imperfections of the methods employed, it remained long unknown that scorbutic disease was prevalent; and it is scarcely yet on record that it existed in seventy per cent. of the sick. If it had been known, it might have been early checked. The remedy was at hand at the very time (January, 1855,) when half the army was dead or sick of it. At a time when the avowed cases at Scutari were reported at 723 admissions to hospital, and 75 deaths, the number now ascertained to have been admitted, suffering under scorbutic disease, was 7761, and the dead were no less than 2253. Such were the errors at a time when a weekly return was published in London of the deaths in the metropolis from all causes, and of the force of each existing disease. The truth is, there are arrangements in London for obtaining and recording the facts; and there is no good reason why the same thing should not be done for an army. It is done in London, not by gathering up from every medical man the notes of his practice, week by week, but by having a method of registration of deaths which furnishes the causes of death. If the same plan, or an analogous one, were instituted in regard to the army at home and abroad, we should soon get far beyond the painful, though necessary, knowledge of how many men have died, to the more fruitful knowledge how to save more from dying, by being duly aware of their dangers.

Thus far, whatever was done at Scutari was by means of the overtasked medical men, each striving to make such returns as he could, amidst pestilence and death, and under a crushing load of incompatible and thankless duties.

Nursing. — Before quitting the review of the Medical Department in the hospital, it is necessary to attend to the all-important business of the nursing of the wounded and sick. Among all the nine departments we are surveying, where is provision made for this nursing?

Regimental Methods. — As long as there is no proper organisation of a General Hospital, each such establishment is, as we have seen, merely a group of regimental hospitals, with as many dispensaries, each containing its small parcels of medicines and instruments, each its own books, and each its own officers, taking the best care they can of their own patients, every one of whom may be suffering under a different malady. To each batch there is a Hospital Sergeant, — the most wonderful man in the army, if he does what is laid upon him. The medical officer and he are supposed to manage the regimental hospital between them; and the sergeant's share is to superintend the wards; to see the patients attended to, and their medicine given, and their diet supplied, with all the variety ordered; to help with the admission returns, and all the other returns, and the accounts; and to look after the washing, the stores, the furniture, the surgery, the medicines, and, in short, whatever has to be taken care of. At no time can one man do all this properly; and what is he to do in a time of epidemic, or a throng of wounded? Some of us have seen the wounded landed at Portsmouth. Though two or three officers had bustled about, and done all they could, what a landing it was! We felt it a disgrace that many of our poor fellows did not know which way to turn themselves, or find anybody to take care of them when they set foot on shore beyond thrusting them into second-class carriages for the hospital, without couch or pillow. Just like this was the way as long as there was no organisation on a large scale, — no preparation for receiving numbers of men under one method, and numbers under another, instead of dealing with them in little heterogeneous groups. But the provision hitherto has been too small for even a regimental hospital, where there should never be fewer than two men; one to take military charge, to attend to the wards and the nursing; to dispense the medicines, and take charge of the surgery; and another to attend to the provisions, the cooking, and the stores, and accounts connected with them, and to the washing. Besides this, there must be orderlies to nurse the sick in proportion to the number of patients.

These officials being needed at all events, which would answer best, — to have a dozen sets of them put down, with their regimental circumstances about them, in a vast hospital like the general one at Scutari; or to organise a body of persons with a view to the extent of the hospital? Instead of repeating what we have already seen, let us look at the nursing alone.

Certain men of the Medical Staff Corps are supposed to be fitted for this kind of duty; and it is certainly a step gained to have men appointed to it, instead of being fetched and carried between military and hospital duty at random. But they have no medical or surgical training, so that that they cannot dress a blister, nor put on a bandage properly, nor get ready the surgeon's instruments, nor stop a hæmorrhage. One was found innocently trying to make a patient eat his poultice; and others stand by while the overtasked surgeon spreads a dressing on lint, or measures out the most simple and ordinary medicine; — moreover, the best men will not be chosen for this service while the choice rests with the military officer. Under no circumstances have the Medical Staff Corps, or orderlies generally, in the hospitals been found adequate to the pressure of a throng of sick or wounded; and it is rarely that they can afford the assistance and support which physicians and surgeons have a right to require from the nurses under their command. At Scutari, the pressure was so alarming, that Government sent out a body of female nurses at one week's notice, under the charge of Miss Nightingale. The chronicles of the time relate who they were, and how they went, and how they were welcomed on the Continent *en route;* but we do not need to turn to those records to refresh our memories. We do not forget, and we never shall forget, any of the circumstances.

The Female Nurses. — These nurses and the wounded from Inkerman met at Scutari, the former arriving there on the eve of the battle.

Hospital Discipline.— What they found in the way of accommodation and management we have seen. The state of things in their own particular province was this. There was no hospital discipline, in the proper sense of the word. This does not mean that there was fighting in the wards, or that the authorities were treated with disrespect; but that, one way or another, orders were not obeyed, — practice did not follow precept. In the camp the discipline of the men in military matters was all that could be desired. When orders were issued, they were understood, each man knew what to do, and every man did it, as a matter of course. Thus the authorities could depend on all below them, and the professional duty was done in the best possible manner. The high character of the British soldier is the result of this intelligence, spirit, and habit of obedience, in combination. The same result would have followed in hospital if the means and method had been the same: but the intelligence was wanting. The orderlies did not understand their business, and the sick had no conception of a discipline in the ward as thorough as that of the ranks. They did not know that their own lives, and those of their comrades, depended upon it. The nurses therefore entered among a mob of sufferers, and had to establish discipline in the wards before they could hope to do much more. They did it by their own example of instant and constant obedience to orders; and by introducing order into their own province.

There ought to have been some one charged with maintaining hospital discipline; but there was no one whose special business it was. The ward-master or hospital-sergeant was hard at work about other affairs. The orderlies had never been trained to clean and air the wards. Their ways (and each took his own way) "would have made a house-maid laugh," we are told. "The patients undid it all, and it had to be done over again." It was all a chance whether medicine or food was taken. If the surgeon gave the medicine with his own hand, the patient had it; if not, he took it or left it, as he chose, or was able. When the meals came, the stronger patients who could feed themselves got some; but the weak, and especially those who could not rise in bed or feed themselves, lay too often unfed. Messes of arrowroot and wine were seen standing cold and stiff by the bedside of a sinking sufferer till they was thrown away at night. The orderlies appeared not to know the importance of the patients, in certain surgical cases, being laid in particular positions; and it was usually neglected. So were many bed-sores. Unless the men asked to be washed, they were left dirty; their wounds were not cleansed and dressed with the simple dressings which nurses are in civil hospitals expected to undertake. Poultices were left on when they were cold and hard, and then not washed off. Some patients were up who ought not to have left their beds; and others were in bed who ought to have been up. Some slipped out of the way to smoke a sly pipe, in draughts or bad smells. The introduction of female Nurses brought much immediate comfort: but it was more important as ultimately producing something of hospital discipline. It was no small matter to see them enter the wards with supplies of hot broth and arrowroot, with wine and cooling drinks, giving what was wanted or longed for, just at the right moment. It was no small matter to get rid of everything dirty, and have everything brought in clean. It was no small matter to have the medicine regularly administered, and the sores quickly and gently dressed. It was no small matter to every man to know that a careful eye was upon him. But the grand achievement was the organisation of hospital management. The idea was conveyed into the minds of the persons concerned, and the practice itself was established in the hospitals.

The object of all hospital management in the army is that the commands of the military authority should be obeyed by the well, and those of the medical authorities by the well and the sick. A head nurse, with orderlies under her directions, to do the cleaning, fetching, carrying, and other nursing offices as they became qualified, would make each ward a place of order, quietness, and comfort, where no patient would be neglected, and the doctors' skill would have something like fair play.

The Nurses' kitchens, for the preparation of sick diets, were an important aid to the doctors at Scutari. They made requisitions on those kitchens for extra diets and medical comforts for hundreds of patients for months together, with perfect certainty that the invalids would be duly nourished. The objects of the surgeons were further met by clean linen and other stores being supplied by the nurses; difficulties and privations disappeared, assistance was always at hand, and directions were obeyed.

Confusion of Authorities.—We have now seen how the Medical Department was hampered by its relation to the Purveyor's, which was itself perpetually confounded with the Commissariat. It seems hopeless to attempt to make out the real distinction between the two departments, in regard to supplying the hospitals in the East; and the only clear thing was that Purveyors had no sufficient instructions to produce. Next comes the Engineer. He could do nothing but on the requisition of persons more fit to be under his orders on the particular points in question, than to command him. He could take no measures for ventilation, for instance, without the authority of the Commandant or the Quartermaster-General; or, in an indirect way, the Chief Medical Officer, or the Purveyor. He could not provide a due water supply without authority; and yet, as to both air and water, he ought to be the best judge of the whole group. It was his business to have the kitchens in good order; and yet he could not do it but on the requisition of one authority, countersigned by another. When all seemed ready for the necessary work of building stores, he could not proceed for want of funds, a difficulty under which the Commandant was himself labouring, in regard to repairing the Scutari barracks. As soon as the impediment was known in England, Government gave power to our Ambassador at the Porte to speed the work. He endeavoured in vain to get the Turks to do it; and at last the necessary money was advanced to the Engineer from a private source. This is a specimen of the way of going on. Thus helpless was the Engineer about repairing the aqueduct (in which lay the dead horse before spoken of) and the quays, and about getting any work done at all, which he accomplished only by employing Greek labourers to a great extent, and at great risk, and at a later period by the encouragement and with the assistance of the Sanitary Commission. During the whole term he was harassed by an undefined responsibility; sometimes left without orders, and sometimes checked from above, while his subordinates shirked their responsibilities, and threw them all on him; sometimes losing his best helpers by sickness, and never finding any efficient aides supplied in their place; perplexed moreover by contradictory orders at the most critical times. Such was the fourth of the nine departments at Scutari.

The Adjutant-General's business was, as has been said above, to help, on all occasions, by affording fatigue parties for every conceivable purpose. It was he who had also to preserve military discipline. His parties helped to bring the sick and wounded ashore, and carry them to the hospitals, but the Quartermaster-General was charged with the duty of depositing them in their right places. It does not appear why such an authority should ever enter a hospital, which cannot possibly want him if it is properly governed; but his deputy saw the patients landed, sending up boat-loads of them to one hospital till it was full, and then to another, but occasionally suffering from a lapse of memory which sent an additional boat-load to a place already full. If the Engineer had been directed to make a pier between the two great hospitals, nearly all the confusion would have been saved; and many a painful scene, with dismal processions of stretchers carried "by unwilling Turks, or feeble convalescents," through the dreary wintry weather, would have been spared. Thus, this one of the nine departments seems to have been merely unnecessary and perplexing.

Next, the Contractor, who supplied the articles needed by the Commissariat. Here is further confusion about the supplies. The Purveyor can do nothing with the Contractor, because the Commissariat stands between. In our hospitals at home the Purveyor deals with the Contractor, and has an interest in seeing that he discharges his duty. At Scutari, the Purveyor desired this, but had not the power; whereas the Commissariat had the power, but was not in a position to care about the fact. These, with the Paymaster and Commandant, make up the nine departments.

Organisation proposed. — Thus were the General Hospitals at Scutari managed,— we cannot say organised. Now let us see how a General Hospital should be organised, according to the Royal Commissioners. They had before them the most extensive and the soundest materials ever offered for a judgment on this point; they have devoted their most earnest attention to it; they feel confidence in their view; and one reason why they may well do so is that their view coincides with Miss Nightingale's. After the experience of the Scutari hospitals, no one will question the value of her opinion as to how that kind of institution should be managed.

Preliminary Conditions. — The conditions of success with that kind of institution must be attended to before the official corps can be described.

1. It must be taken for granted that some sanitary

agency will exist in connection with the army:—that, wherever the troops go or rest, there shall be a department charged with the care of the wholesomeness of their surroundings. There must be an Army-Works Corps, or a Pioneers' Corps, to work under Engineers for purposes of health and convenience. These arrangements are necessary everywhere, and cannot be dispensed with where hospitals exist.

2. There must be General Hospitals enough, at home and abroad, if any one is to do its duty satisfactorily. There must be two or more in England, where all the officials, from the Governor to the humblest attendant, shall have practised their duties. There must be a General Hospital at the base of operations. Regimental hospitals will remain as they are,—best for their particular purpose, and indispensable. When a siege is in progress, or the army is in winter quarters, some regimental hospitals may, and will be modified so as to make a central hospital on the spot for the temporary need.

3. In order to have all necessary resources at hand, there must be a Depôt within reach of the General Hospital, with a Quarter-Master-General's store, out of which the deficiencies of the soldiers' kit, arms, and accoutrements may be made up. But the depôt must not be under the same roof with the hospital. It is better a mile off, at least. It might furnish guards to the hospital, but cannot be under the same command.

4. As to the interior of the hospital; it is necessary that there should be a body of men trained to hospital duty,—properly taught to keep the place and its inmates in a clean and comfortable state, and to wait on the doctors and the patients. There must also be an establishment of Female Nurses, duly recognised as having their proper business in the hospital, and authorised to do that business and no more.

The patients must be simply patients, and not soldiers; subject to the authorities of the hospital while they remain there, and returning to their military character, and their own officers, when they go out recovered.

These reasonable and necessary conditions being admitted, the government of a General Hospital becomes a much simpler affair than it has ever hitherto appeared. The Report of the Commissioners, and the Evidence on which it was grounded, furnish proposals which we must hope to see carried into effect.

Offices few and distinct.—The organisation is required for the sanitary welfare of the hospital; for its government; for the medical care of the inmates; and for the supply of their wants. These being the objects, there can be no occasion for nine departments of office.

Whatever is true about the necessity of sanitary care in the establishment of a camp applies with the utmost force to the founding and care of a hospital. The sanitary charge ought not to be devolved on the

Governor, any more than the purchase of provisions, or the superintendence of the washing. There is plenty of employment, we are told, for a sanitary officer in a General Hospital: and his department must be directly responsible to the Governor, like all but the medical, which is subordinate to its own chief.

The Governor.—THE GOVERNOR must be chosen, in the first place, for his administrative ability, which is a matter of more importance than his being a soldier, a civilian, a physician, or of any other description. The office must be considered a civil one, whether the Governor be a soldier or a doctor, or neither. There need be nothing military about the whole establishment, except that one or more officers from the Adjutant-General's Department should be on the spot to conduct the discipline of the convalescents about to return to the army, and to see that they are properly equipped when they leave the hospital. The patients are sick as men, not as soldiers; and the nearer the management approaches to that of civil hospitals, the better it will be.

The Governor should be appointed by the War Office; and fitness ought to be the sole consideration. The function is a peculiar one; and if the range of several professions is thrown open for the choice, the obligation to choose for fitness alone is imperative to the last degree. The authority of the office should be equal to that of Governor of a fortress. Every one would be subject to the Governor, except in the one department of medical administration; and the Governor would be responsible solely to the War Office, or to the Commander-in-Chief. He must reside in the hospital, and be constantly acquainted with all its departments. The total organisation would rest on him. All others would be working in their respective departments; it would be his business to keep the whole system going in order and harmony; and his decision would be indisputable, except in provided cases where an appeal would lie to the War Office or the Commander-in-Chief.

Here we have one official combining the functions of three under the old system;—the Commandant, Adjutant-General, and Quartermaster-General.

Chief Medical Officer.—Next comes the CHIEF MEDICAL OFFICER, selected also for fitness alone. His business would be to take the entire charge of the medical officers, medicines, and management of the sick. When the doctors and their staff, from the *chef* to the humblest dresser and dispenser, are relieved from all but professional duties, the time will have arrived for a great expansion of professional science and skill. Hitherto all has been confusion in these great establishments, and there has been nothing like that amount of medical lore resulting from so vast a practice that there ought to have been. The desultory character of the observations, the confusion in the assortment of diseases, and the misleading nomenclature which still subsists, will all be in the way of correction when the medical officers have ceased to be clerks and purveyors, and are enabled to practise, to study, and to conduct the studies of their subordinates, according to their rightful and reasonable claims.

The Steward.—THE STEWARD comes next; the official charged with the care of Supply. He would be responsible to the Governor alone, and would receive his orders and powers from no other quarter. There would be an end of the cumbrous system of requisitions, and of extra-diet lists. After due inquiry and consultation, according to the peculiarities of each case of a hospital established abroad, a fixed scale of supply would be agreed upon, for the guidance of the Steward, who would give out whatever was wanted, on the Governor's written authority. By the institution of a more varied dietary, a vast amount of special ordering would be spared; the stores wanted for an establishment containing a certain number of persons, once ascertained, would be regularly procured if one department was charged with the business, instead of the work and the powers being divided; and this would be the Steward's business. He would receive the Governor's orders to provide specified supplies, and would be empowered to compel contractors to fulfil their bargains, or to purchase at their expense whatever they have failed to supply. He would be responsible for the care of the stores, and under obligation to report their amount periodically.

The Treasurer.—THE TREASURER follows. His

function would be to provide funds, to make payments under the Governor's order, to keep the accounts, and to examine the Steward's accounts and vouchers, before they are sent home for audit.

The Superintendent of Service. — There remains the Orderly Service of the establishment. There should be a Captain of that service. He might be a soldier, a civilian, or a doctor, but must have decided administrative ability. The whole body of attendants must be under him, as a regiment is under its commanding officer, his authority extending to the whole interior economy which is not occupied by the Medical and the Steward's departments. The orderlies, cooks, washers, and linen store keepers would be under his control; the furniture, bedding, clothes, and supplies of all kinds would be his charge; and he would be responsible for the condition and comfort of the patients.

These offices seem to include everything needed; and the distribution of duties and powers obviates the confusion, awkwardness, and perplexity which paralysed even the ablest officials at the most critical moments. There are plenty of large establishments, — and not a few large hospitals, — in the civilised world which are well governed and administered without any desperate difficulty. The thing can be done in any part of the world where our soldiers are ever likely to go; and it must be done. We have had enough of vain struggles to stretch Regimental Hospitals beyond their capacity; and of excessive mortality as a characteristic of General Hospitals. We have learned what Regimental Hospitals can and cannot do; and that a General Hospital may be made favourable to recovery; and what is wanted to make it so. Having learned these things, we must see that they are put in practice at once, in time of peace, and to such an extent as to keep us always ready for any call of war. We must have one, two, or three General Hospitals at home, organised in the best known manner, and used as schools for the training of officials, and especially for the formation of bodies of nurses, male and female.

In the last war the lesson given was one which should not only be remembered, but understood to the very bottom. The preparations at Scutari being inadequate to an astounding degree, the misery was such as to be intolerable now in the retrospect; and the mortality was only short of total loss of our army. When the state of things mended, it was not by means of any substantive reform which we can point to now as a security against the same calamity recurring. The soldiers were saved by a peremptory breaking through all rules, and the most lavish expenditure of money ever witnessed in our military history. While a miserable network of rules and forms had trammelled everybody, for the avowed purpose of checking expenditure in the minutest particulars, hundreds and thousands of our costly trained soldiers died in heaps. Thousands of young and raw soldiers were sent to fill their places, and died off faster still. It was intolerable. All obstructions were overthrown, —all impeding forms broken through; and then occurred the most prodigious waste ever perpetrated by rational people. The waste was itself rational. The remnant of our soldiers was saved by the most rapid pouring out of help and comfort that the national heart and soul could achieve. There were agents, happily, whose energy and daring were equal to the crisis. They have shown us what could be done, at last, and they instruct us now as to what remains to be done. We cannot run such a risk twice; it would be a grave evil to permit such an abeyance of discipline, and a sin to countenance such extravagance again. But these evils are not even yet guarded against. If we do not insist on the reforms which we all approve, we shall find some day that we have slid back into the old ineffective methods which have cost us so many pangs and tears, and so much blood and treasure. We have no Sanitary Department in the army yet; no Model Hospital; no certainty that our Commissariat is equal to all probable calls upon it; no clear connection between the provision of stores and the soldiers' enjoyment of them. We are not yet putting into practice in peace the lessons we received with so much horror in war. We must look to it. We have several lost years to account for already. We might have been in easy training by this time: but where are our New Departments? — where is our improved Army-medical Education? — where are our General Hospitals, with their great medical schools, and statistical offices? — where is our trained Medical Staff Corps, fit to undertake hospital nursing in an adequate way? — and where is our body of selected, instructed, disciplined Female Nurses, who should be the sick soldier's best reliance when overtaken by the casualties of war? Whatever may be the excuses for our delay, there can be no adequate reason. The need is greater than any possible impediment. The growl of the war tempest is heard on the horizon; and we are not ready. If misfortune happens, — if one soldier dies through our dilatoriness, what shall we say?

CHAP. VIII.

RESTORATION.

THE long lane had its turning at last. The wounded from Inkerman who survived the first crowding, the hospital gangrene, and other causes of mortality, could not forget, if they were to live a thousand years, the first approaches of comfort, the first sensations of convalescence. Too many of them died, in spite of the resistance to death set up by devoted doctors and nurses. Some were kept alive, when given over from the severity of their wounds,—kept alive by watchful hands administering spoonfuls of nourishment through the night, and strengthening them for surgical treatment in the morning. Others were long in hospital, and not a few were invalided home; and, finally, more and more went back to the siege of Sebastopol. If these men honour their nurses, not less do the nurses honour most of the men. The courage of our soldiers was never doubted,—their valour in the battle-field; but it could never have been known but by being witnessed what was their pluck in hospital,—their indomitable patience as they lay on their beds of pain. Whatever their anguish, they could consider others. Among thousands of them, scarcely one uttered an oath, or any other word that could give pain to their nurses. They were grateful for every wish to serve them. They never flinched from the duty which cost them so dear, and gave up limb and life as if they themselves did not estimate the sacrifice; and after such an act as that, they accepted the smallest aid as so much bounty. It is no wonder that some of the best hearts and minds among us were eager to save and serve such men. On the other hand, it is no wonder that such men felt, in the depths of their hearts, what was done for them by the Commissioners sent out from England, and the Ladies who ministered to them day and night. When comfort began to creep through the place, and the convalescent more and more outnumbered the dead, sufferers and nurses began to reap their reward. To us, who merely read of what has long been past, the sensation of relief is very strong.

Quietness and Comfort.—The Sanitary Commission came out, and set ventilation and cleansing going on everywhere. Openings were made for air; foul smells were first carried off, and then put an end to, and the interior of the hospitals was "scrupulously clean." The Depôt was removed from the Barrack Hospital, with its noise, and its crowd, and its military habits and associations; and the quietness befitting a habitation of the sick was established. By this time every patient lay in clean sheets, and had always a change of linen. By this time everyone was secure against being forgotten, or his wound passed by in the scramble of numbers. He was attended to as his turn came round,—his wound dressed, his medicine given, and his extra meal brought, good and punctual. By this time books and newspapers, among other luxuries, had arrived, and the nurses were not too busy to spare minutes, and even hours, in finding for the patients the particular volumes they wished for. Huts for the convalescents were put up in the yard of the Barrack Hospital: and one of these was allowed to be made a Reading-room for the men. A private hand stocked it with books, maps, prints, newspapers, and writing materials, and a non-commissioned officer took charge of it. It was open at all hours. The men wrote their letters there; and it was filled with readers all day long. It was as quiet and orderly as the Library of the British Museum. As it was prophesied that the men would sell the writing paper for drink, some attention was paid to the quantity which disappeared; and it was found to correspond with the amount of letters sent to Miss Nightingale to be stamped. As some of the paper given out in the wards disappeared (not sold by either patient or orderly), the sick who could not leave their beds were supplied from the Reading-room, and the paper was thenceforth used for correspondence. What a change in the scene,—when every patient's wishes and tastes could be considered, and their minds cared for as effectually as their bodies! A death in the ward became rarer and rarer; the new patients from the Crimea were less and less dirty and wretched in appearance, and less sunk in strength, showing an improved condition of affairs at the seat of war: and they had now every chance in hospital.

Mortality, first and last. — The change in a year, in both Camp and Hospital, affords a lesson which ought to preserve all future armies. Under one method of proceeding, 18,000 men died, who, under another method, would have lived. One end of this wrong method was working in the camp, and the other at Scutari; and men were dying all along the line. On the Black Sea, within the space of 300 miles, nearly seventy-five per 1000 died out of 13,093 sent from the camp. In January, 1855, ten died on the passage to every hundred received at Scutari. Of those who arrived in the Bosphorus, more than four hundred per cent. per annum, and at Koulali, more than six hundred per cent., died in hospital. No pesthouse could be more fatal than the Camp, the Transport, and the Hospital. During the first seven months in the Crimea, the deaths from disease alone, without reckoning the genuine casualties of war, were at the rate of sixty per cent. per annum of the whole force. During the last six months of the war, the mortality among the troops was only two-thirds what it is at home. So much for the Camp! As for the Hospitals, it is enough to say, that the mortality among the patients there scarcely exceeded that of the healthy Guards at home.

In February, 1855, two men died of every five at Scutari, and one of every two at Koulali. By June, the mortality had sunk to a nineteenth part of this proportion.

Occupations.—We heard a good deal about intemperance still. It was a subject of grief and shame to us in England that soldiers whom we had honoured for valour, fortitude, patience,—in short, for heroism,—were weak in that direction, and brought disgrace on their name and fame. It was painful to hear that soldiers from the depôt bought liquors at the Greek wine-shops, and supplied them secretly to the patients, sending up bottles by a string let down from a window. It was painful to hear that patients, who had been nursed with care and anxiety, and dismissed full of gratitude, were brought back on stretchers, poisoned with the infamous local drink, against which they had been emphatically warned. But this evil was overcome, like all the rest. In August, the Inkerman Coffee-house (as it was called) was opened at Scutari by the benevolence of private contributors and managers. It was a large hut, provided with refreshments, newspapers, prints and games. When it had been opened two months, the last commandant at Scutari put a stop to the sale of spirits there and elsewhere. The spirits were hunted out and destroyed, and drunkenness was at an end. Every drunken soldier was thenceforth sure of detection, exposure, and punishment. The streets were patrolled, and every soldier of every rank was challenged after dusk. There was no dulness from this change, but quite the contrary. The men were never so well amused before.

During the last few months there were four Schools. Schoolmasters were sent out from England for the Garrison School, and a magnificent hut was erected for it. The lectures were so crowded that the men took the doors off the hinges to enable more to hear. Singing-classes were formed; and the members were allowed to sing in the garrison chapel. The strong men played foot-ball, and other muscular games; and the weakly enjoyed chess and dominoes. We remember how the Queen and the Duchess of Kent sent out supplies of books, newspapers, and games. One great amusement was the little theatre got up by the men, where a great deal of fun went forward, without any disorder.

During the last months of the war, the sick from Balaclava were fewer and fewer, and they arrived in a better state. The wards in the hospitals had long ceased to be over-crowded, and were more and more scantily occupied. There was comfort everywhere, and leisure to keep up the style of comfort. In every former war it had been said that to send men into a General Hospital was to send them to death. In this war it had long appeared only too true. But it was now proved beyond dispute that a General Hospital may be made as healthy an establishment as any abode whatever. It should never be forgotten that the mortality among the sick there scarcely exceeded that of the healthy Guards at home. This carries us over to the camp in the Crimea, where, as may well be repeated, the mortality among the troops was now only two-thirds what it is at home.

Improvement in Camp.—It is a satisfaction in which we may indulge, to look round the plateau before Sebastopol, and see the contrast between the soldier's life at the opening of 1855 and a year later. The material of the troops was finer the first year than the second. The thousands who died in that terrible autumn and winter were picked men and trained soldiers; mature in years and frame, exercised in their profession, and originally selected as the healthiest men under the best conditions of health. The reinforcements sent out were, to a considerable extent, young; even immature, inexperienced, only beginning to understand discipline; raw levies, in short; whereas those we had lost were a genuine British force of the highest quality, as their conduct in the field showed, to the conviction of all the world. Now that these were buried, what was life in the Crimea to their survivors?

Hospitals.—We saw before what was done to regenerate Balaclava. There was a General Hospital there; a large stone building, for which everything was done that the conditions of the case admitted; but it served better as a transit hospital than as a place of recovery for the sick, and was latterly so used. The Castle Hospital was finely placed on a height above the sea, well supplied with air, on a dry soil, and commanding a supply of pure water. The establishment consisted of huts, some of a better and some of an inferior construction; but such improvements were introduced, by raising the ridge pieces and making openings, so as to ventilate the interior, and moderating the heat of the sun, that an extraordinary proportion of recovery was obtained for the wounded and sick. It was occupied chiefly by wounded, of whom only three per cent. died; and, of sick and wounded together, only three and a quarter per cent. were lost. There are few instances on record of such success in hospital management. The Monastery Hospital was a healthy one too; but it was occupied by convalescents chiefly, and by ophthalmia cases from the front. One other, unfavourably situated, was gradually used for other purposes; and very few sick remained in it during the last winter. Except those few, the sick in General Hospitals were on high and dry ground, with space, pure air and comfort all about them, and every chance for recovery. The Regimental Hospitals—groups of huts, with here and there a tent, scattered where they were wanted, were prodigiously improved through the advanced experience of the medical officers and their increased command of means.

As for the soldiers generally, they were in a condition of health such as is seldom seen even at home, except among men of the healthiest occupation. If poor Bob's friends in the old village at home could have followed him in his adventures during the war, and have seen him pass through the reeking mists in Bulgaria, and the hot marches in the Crimea, and the cold damps and semi-starvation on the plateau, and the voyage to Scutari, to lie long there in fever, and the difficult recovery, and the return to camp, they would never have expected to see him as he now began to appear. While his old acquaintance, the clerk, the shopman, the policeman at home, were undergoing variations of health according to the liabilities of their calling, he who had sunk lower than any of them was now rising into a condition of robustness such as none of them had ever enjoyed.

Drainage.—He was a good deal employed during the autumn and winter, in the work once so familiar to him,—digging. The Army-Works Corps in the Crimea had done great good to the health of the troops by the drainage which accompanied the railways. Trenches were dug in various directions, to carry off the waters from the works; and the effect was so manifestly good that new energy was imparted to the task, done by the soldiers, of making roads wherever communication went forward; old lines of road were repaired, new ones were made, and the character of the ground required much deep trenching. The watercourses down to the harbour were straightened and improved. The marshy spots shrank and disappeared; the ground became dry and pervious; bad smells died out, and the soldiers showed broad chests, stout arms, and the gait of robust men.

Winter.—Towards the end of October, 1855, a close and thorough survey of the camp was gone through, to ascertain how far due preparation had been made for the winter; and within two months everything was arranged for the splendid sanitary close of the war. No two regiments were exactly alike, it was observed, in the skill with which they made these preparations. Some were hutted in ample time, some in a hurry, and some after the men had begun to suffer from damp and cold. Some had done the trenching better and some worse; some obtained better cookery than others, and stricter order in the canteen. If all had been early and duly trained, so as to equal or excel the best on the plateau, the close might have been more striking even than it was.

Clothing.—As it was, there was health and comfort for every man who chose to deserve it,—apart, of course, from the wounded, and from those who had not entirely recovered from previous illness. An abundance of woollen clothing was distributed in good time. All the officers and the experienced soldiers generally wore it next their skins. Some of the young men did not; and the ordinary consequence was, a liability to the old disorders. Where the surgeons took care that the men wore their flannels properly, there was almost entire freedom from those ailments. Waterproof-jackets and capes saved many lives, the medical officers declare.—The bedding was something very unlike the blanket spread on the mud of a year before. Dry, sufficient, and laid in wholesome huts, it was as good as any man in the camp would have had at home.

Food.—The food was not yet all that it might have been; but the change was prodigious. The soldiers still longed for flour and peas, which were easy of transport, and ought not to have been deficient; but scurvy, and the group of maladies which are all scurvy under different names, had almost entirely disappeared from the army, while they prevailed very seriously in the encampments of our allies, where the management was not so good as ours was now. There was always plenty of food for all our men;—vegetables without stint, and fresh meat three or four times a week, and soft bread, with rice, sugar, coffee (fit for use), tea, pepper, and salt. Salt meat and hard biscuit were still thrown away pretty often, whereas fresh meat and soft bread never were.

Drink.—The worst incident was the spirit-drinking. Half a gill was served out *neat* the first thing in the morning; and the young soldiers, who were least tempted at the outset, soon followed the example of their elders, and drank it off. The natives,—both soldiers and workmen,—either made themselves ill with drinking the new poison, or sold it to our men, who drank the more. After the cessation of the siege the manifest increase of intemperance was brought to the notice of the Commander-in-Chief; a board of officers consulted about it; and the allowance of rum was reduced one half, while that of sugar was doubled. The news of the disgrace and the subsequent improvement reached us at home; but we never derived an impression of such complete reform as was effected at Scutari.

The Canteens.—In some regiments, the officers proved themselves excellent friends to their men by undertaking the trouble of managing the Canteen. They bought the stores, placed them under good care, and had them sold at prices which merely covered the expenses. It need not be explained that the best assortment, and the best quality of articles, might be found at such canteens, at lower prices than elsewhere. Instead of a sixpenny glass of infamous spirit, the men could have at the same cost half a pound of cheese, or two draughts of beer or porter. The most successful management, however, left the strongest impression that the whole system ought to be on a different footing in future. The diet of the soldiers ought to be all found for them; and the canteens should be so stocked, by arrangements between the departments of the service, as to hold out the least temptation to self-indulgence, while supplying the best quality of whatever is sold, at a lower rate than can ever be secured by the chance methods of the camp.

Cookery.—In no respect was the change greater than in the preparation of the food. From some quarter or other a stove had arrived in almost every regimental kitchen. The commanding officer, or friends at a distance, had presented it, to save fuel, and cook dinners for many at once. The economy of cooking on a large scale had become apparent to everybody in the camp; and the devices to do it formed a remarkable spectacle. The camp-kettles were less and less used; and powder cases were resorted to, each of which cooked the rations of forty men or more. In this new receptacle the food could be kept warm for those who returned from duty in the trenches. After the troops had obtained access to Sebastopol, they brought up large boilers, which were a great comfort. When such a boiler was properly fixed, with a fireplace under it, and a powder case built in next to it, for an oven, there was really nothing more to desire. As the men remarked, the fuel which had formerly served a company was now enough for the whole regiment. Two of a company were employed in cooking; and the assistant of one week was the cook of the next.

All took their turns, and thus had a fortnight's practice at a time. Still, there was a distinctive character about the kitchens, which seemed to be under a common method of management. The same varieties in the sense and skill and taste of the men showed themselves here as in other directions. Some kitchens were dirty, smoky, and disgusting, while others, close at hand, were neat, convenient, and appetising, — the difference depending on the way that the men had been trained, or were commanded. The time of hardship was over, however. Those who chose could have comfortable meals.

M. Soyer was conspicuous in the camp. Willing to incite, to instruct, to assist, he was truly a good friend to the soldier, and a powerful contributor to the high average of health which was attained on the plateau. He did not live to see the army fed as we may hope the existing generation may yet see it; but his name must not be forgotten when the story is told of the renovation of our forces in the Crimean war.

The Close of their Duty.—When the troops were in the height of their vigour, and were longing to show what they could do, — they who had never yet been beaten in their days of sickness, hunger, and diminished numbers, — they were told that the war was over. They brought away such stores as they were ordered to convey to the ships; they left behind the greatest mass of shot and shell ever deposited within an equal area, and turned their backs on many warped and broken huts, and the bits of wall, and trench, and oven that had made up a home for them. They left behind the graves of thousands of comrades. The last that remained was a company of the 50th Regiment, which was posted outside of Balaclava, to await the Russian guard. The Russian guard came up; the British turned and marched in with them, saw them place their sentries, exchanged salutes with them, and preceded General Codrington and his staff in going on board H.M.S. Algiers, which brought away the last British soldier from the Crimea.

The Beginning of ours.—This was on the 12th of July, 1856. Nearly three years have elapsed; and how much of our solemn lesson have we put in practice? History has nothing to show that can compare in clearness with the illustration that the Crimean war affords of the results of wisdom and folly in the administration of our military resources. We have seen a complete and undisguised exemplification of the loss and the renovation of our national armies. The lesson cost us 18,000 men, for whose loss our ignorance was answerable. Such an experiment cannot be tried repeatedly by a nation in warfare, as a scientific one by a philosopher in his laboratory; but one would think that we intended it, by our hesitation in practically adopting the instruction. After three years, while we have, and must continue to have, a large army in India, and while the hum and murmur of warfare is growing louder with every shifting wind, what have we done towards renovating and preserving our military strength? We saved the remnant of our soldiers by a total disruption of forms and regulations, and by a wild waste of money. We set to work to learn the right method of preserving our army by means of wise regulations, and that generous economy which proves the best thrift in the end. The right method is ascertained and disclosed, and a few desultory reforms have been instituted; but our system is still unfavourable in a high degree to the health and longevity of the soldier, and there is no approach to completeness in our care of the *physique* of the British army. The thing has to be done. There is no time to lose in doing it. Why is it not done?

This is the question to which we must have an answer before we can recruit our forces to any purpose. If we ever do recruit to such purpose as may be expected of the people of England,—that people so proud to be appealed to *pro rege, lege, grege,*—it will be after that people has made its fair condition, and imposed its solemn behest on the government,—NO MORE LOST ARMIES!

CHAP. IX.

WHAT REMAINS.

Views of the Hour. — THE world is full of warlike propensities at present. No nation can feel secure of a term of peace, long or short. The most restless of our neighbours have a prodigious proportion of soldiery to the area of their territory; whereas England has a prodigious proportion of territory to take care of with a small army. The Continental nations obtain augmentations of force by conscription, under one name or another; whereas our only resource is inducement to volunteers.—This is one view.

It has thus far been universally true, that the dangers of the military profession arise less from the enemy than from the incidents of the mode of life in which the enemy have no concern. The killed and wounded form a very small proportion of the sufferers by a campaign. Disease from exposure, fatigue, and want, is far more fatal than shot, shell, and bayonet; and when disease arrives in the form of epidemics, the troops in fact sustain at once the horrors of war and pestilence; and the two classes of evils ought not to be mixed up together, and laid at the door of war. All the armies of our time have been seen suffering under the evils of disease, whatever their fortunes in conflict. In the late Russian war, all the combatants pined and perished, in greater or smaller proportion,— the Russians the worst, but all very bitterly. We, for our part, have ascertained that this largest and bitterest portion of the fatality and suffering of warfare is avoidable. We have ascertained what average of mortality from disease ought not to be exceeded. We have ascertained that if that average were not exceeded, warfare would cost us fewer soldiers than we have been accustomed to lose in peace; all apprehension of an inconvenient drain of our stout young citizens would be at an end, a certain moderate amount of recruiting would sustain a much larger force than has been yet contemplated; or, in other words, a smaller re-inforcement than has yet been calculated on, would sustain our military strength at the desired point.— This is another view.

The actual military strength of any country depends more on the quality of the individual soldiers than on any other consideration whatever. Every influence which impairs the soldier's health and security tends to lower his quality; and, conversely, every exertion of knowledge, skill, justice, and kindness which contributes to his welfare, and testifies to his value, tends to elevate his quality. While the profession has been so hazardous as to be considered a reckless calling, reckless, floating, purposeless, ignorant or disreputable men offer themselves, and are heard of afterwards as the deserters who shame us by their numbers. If our system were at this moment organised on the principles of military hygiene, our accession of strength would soon be duplicate, and much more. Our existing soldiers would, for the most part, fairly live out their time in the world: the new comers would live on in like manner: and those new comers would be men who enter the army for some better reason than that they do not know what else to do with themselves, or, to escape from some evil at home, will take their chance of danger abroad. The quality of our best soldiers before Sebastopol is a fair measure of what our army generally might be if its high quality were taken for granted in our arrangements for the life of the army. How this superiority is the same thing as an economy of force, needs no detailed explanation. And, again, it cannot be necessary to do more than suggest that, from the moment when we adopt in practice the principles and arts of military hygiene, we become the equals or superiors of the most imposing military powers whose forces are not so husbanded.—This is another view.

It does not appear that these truths are disputed. We have employed a Royal Commission to ascertain and state them clearly for us. We have found them extremely interesting, and full of promise. We have admitted that the result is in our own hands. We take for granted that all will be right henceforth. But we cannot rely on this unless we see the thing done. We cannot even be certain that we are not at this moment edging away from the arrangements which ought to have been in vigorous operation long before this time. If three years have been allowed to pass since the evacuation of the Crimea without our having utilised the experience we got there, what can we hope from the next three years? This is the question which the people of England, military, naval, and civilian, must urge in an effectual way.

Practical Aims and Recommendations.—The Report of the Commissioners affords all necessary instruction as to the precise points to be aimed at.—Following the course of my narrative, I may review these points in some such order as this.

I. *Hygiene a Separate Department.*—The principles and art of Military Hygiene must be brought into operation for the maintenance of our national defence by the preservation of our soldiery.

The care of the healthy being one thing, and the care of the sick another, both must be specially provided for. That is, there must be both a Sanitary and a Medical Department supplied to the army. Both must be represented in Council, and both must be responsible in action.

II. *The Medical Council.*—The Council which takes charge of the *physique* of the army should consist of the Director-General of the Medical Department, and three Councillors; one medical, one sanitary, and one statistical. Each of these three would give his opinion in writing, and submit questions on occasion; each would manage the routine business of his own function; but the ultimate decision on all questions before the Board, and the responsibility of decision, would rest with the Director-General.

III. *Concert between Departments.*—The concert which is necessary between the Military and Medical Departments, and between both these and the Sanitary must be secured by express arrangement and regulation; whereby the due supremacy may remain, as it ought, with the military authority, while the lives of soldiers may not be thrown away through timidity, misunderstanding, or collision of authorities. The advisers should know when to point out the dangers of the site, and the condition of the sick, while the commanding officer remains the judge how far to admit considerations of health or sickness into his plans of the hour.

The same concert must be secured between the military and medical officers of the regiment as in the larger instance of the army generally; and by the same means:—by the clear and definite prescription of each department. While the sanitary charge of the army has been appointed to nobody, but attributed sometimes to the commander, sometimes to the

Quarter-master-General, and sometimes to the medical *chef*, who, at the same time, had no authority, the health of the army could not be provided for. The departments, then, and the responsibility, must be so clearly defined as to admit of concert and undivided authority in regard to the sanitary arrangements of the army, at home and abroad.

IV. *Lodgment of the Sanitary Charge.*—Then occurs the grave consideration whether the sanitary charge of the army should be appointed to others than the medical officers. Of the special quality of the science and art there is no doubt, nor, consequently, of the special administration of the function. The only question is whether it can and ought to be joined with the medical function. The decision to which the reforming authorities incline is that the Medical Department may undertake sanitary functions on certain conditions and not otherwise; on condition, that is, that a sanitary official, and also one for hospitals, and one for statistics, is admitted to the Director-General's Council; and that the proposed Medical School is brought into full action.

A step in the right direction has been taken by the appointment of Mr. Alexander to be Director-General of the Medical Department: but the Medical Council is not yet granted. It is perhaps the most important deficiency that remains. As to the Medical School, a small beginning already exists at Chatham.

V. *Medical Education.*—The army physician and

surgeon must have a special training, if the troops are to have a fair chance. The existing medical education of civilian doctors, will be indispensable, with the large additions that the Commissioners have pointed out: and the process of examination must be more trustworthy and effectual than it is at present. The examination for the East India Medical Service is indicated as affording a good model. Nowhere is there at present any means of obtaining an adequate education in military surgery; for the lectures at Edinburgh and Dublin afford theoretical instruction only, and are actually of less value than the general medical and surgical study which they intercept. The school for study at Chatham is a mere hint of what is needed, and altogether inadequate to the requirements of the service. There is no staff of professors; there are no arrangements for the students remaining till they are qualified. No clinical instruction is given by the bed-side; and no instruction in sanitary science is afforded at all.

The requisite Military Medical Education must be given in connection with a Model General Hospital; and this leads us on to the next great requisite, viz:—

VI. *General Hospital and School.* — A Model General Hospital, with as many more as are necessary.

We have seen the results of our crude knowledge and judgment in regard to hospitals; the invariable failure of Regimental hospitals when forced beyond their natural and necessary function; the hopelessness of agglomerating them to supply the place of a General Hospital; and the beneficial and wholly manageable character of General Hospitals, when properly organised. These facts are proved, beyond all danger of dispute. The practical consequences remain.

In every war, there must be General Hospitals. They cannot be established and worked without immediate and constant command of experience, knowledge and habit. We cannot have good hospitals abroad unless we have been accustomed to them at home. We cannot have good hospitals in war unless we have had them in peace. We must have one at home, at once, and perfectly organised on the most perfect principles. The intention was to make Netley serve these purposes; but the Report and Evidence exhibit good and abundant reasons why this cannot be. Neither the position of Netley Hospital, nor its construction, nor its sanitary conditions, nor the kind of patients it will receive, will at all answer the purposes of a Model Hospital and Military Medical School. Acute cases will be rarely seen there, because the place is far from any garrison; and this is enough. There are other reasons, many and strong, against appointing Netley for the purposes of training in hospital management and practice; but one is as good as more; and another site ought to be immediately fixed on for an establishment of the highest class, with its attendant libraries, museum, model-rooms, and means of thorough education for students, accumulation of experience for the future generation of practitioners, and organised care and treatment of the patients.

In connexion with this primary need are the collateral needs of which I have already spoken;—first, a reform in the method of administering General Hospitals; second, a provision of trained Military Nurses, like the present Medical Staff Corps, but properly taught and exercised in the art of tending the wounded and sick; and third, an order of Female Nurses, taught and trained to act in General Hospitals (not Regimental) as they do in civil hospitals, and in the naval one at Haslar. A certain proportion of female nurses to the wards of a General Hospital, or to the number of patients in them, ought to be at command, at home and abroad, from this time forward.

VII. *Army Medical Department.*—When the report of the Commissioners appeared, it was impossible for any person out of the profession (or perhaps in it) to understand with any clearness the rules of the Medical Department of the army, or the status of any member of it. A deep dissatisfaction pervaded the department at the uncertainty and insufficiency of honour and reward, and the dubious relations of the members to each other, to their military companions, and society at large. In this direction a great deed has been done; a beneficent consequence has grown out of the labours of the Commissioners. The warrant for the Army Medical Department, issued last autumn, is a kind of charter to the department. It simplifies and diminishes ranks; it regulates promotion by intelligible rules; it improves the financial position of army physicians and surgeons; and it establishes them in a better relation with their military comrades, giving them a definite rank on intellectual grounds which may counterbalance the *prestige* of military distinction, and enable non-combatants to win a position in that peculiar society in which rank is the highest of rewards. We owe it to General Peel and the Horse Guards that the army medical profession is now an attractive one to men of spirit, instead of a most vexatious and discouraging one. If the other recommendations of the Commissioners had been equally well carried out, our military strength and welfare would have been by this time secure.

VIII. *Organisation.*—That particular class of sanitary reforms which relates to Barracks is apparently well urged forwards. From week to week we read of barracks being improved, drained, ventilated, supplied with baths, with reading, or eating, or working rooms; and especially of a reduction of numbers in certain areas, and re-distribution of the inmates. There is more variety in the diet; more sense in the methods of clothing; greater variety of occupation and exercise. It seems to be seriously intended to practise the soldiers in field-works, and in the arts of camp life. There can be no doubt of our troops being now far better prepared for war than at any time prior to the hard lessons in the Crimea. The thing further wanted is that every advance should be secured by the well-grounded establishment of a complete system, in which every individual should know his own place and his own duty; and duty should be simplified to the utmost by the machinery of a perfect organisation.

So far from this making men into machines, it has precisely the opposite effect. The way to make men into machines is to implicate them with a great burden of forms and rules, planned for small purposes of economy, and ending in enormous failure and waste. Under a good organisation of Supply, for instance, each man in each department is responsible for getting some definite thing done. Under a bad system he is responsible only for calling upon somebody else to do it. The thing is not done; the men are not fed, or physicked, or what not; and those who should do it are put out and helpless. Something must be done; and so rules and forms are burst through by some bold hand: then each does what seems best in his own eyes, and waste ensues, too late to repair the more grievous waste from deficiency. The departments of Supply are hardly within the range of this final chapter; and I will say no more about them than to remind the reader that when the Commissariat had provided vast stores of food and clothing, and brought them to the Crimea, thousands of soldiers died of destitution nevertheless. The food and clothing were almost within sight: but they were not within reach; and they might as well have been in the Thames as at Balaclava. There was a hitch in the organisation. A department was wanted to bring the men and the supplies together; to bring (as was said) the food into their mouths, and the clothes upon their backs. Whether this kind of consideration comes under any sanitary head or not, it must be attended to, if we are to have and to keep an army fit to guard our empire.

Opening the Way. — It is natural for everybody to speculate on the causes of the delay which chafes all good citizens, — soldiers and civilians, men and women, peers and peacemen. It is asked, far and wide, "Who stops the way?" The good will of the sovereign is believed in on solid grounds. Two Secretaries of State have signified their approbation of the reforms recommended by the Commissioners, and the Commander-in-chief is regarded as the soldiers' friend. The obstruction is supposed to lie lower down. Change is abhorred in Government offices. This is a general truth, which it is now proposed in some quarters to make the ground of a Commission of Inquiry in this particular case. The question whether reason and right, justice and mercy, the sovereign, the people, the Parliament, and the army of England, are to be slighted, tampered with, and set aside, when insisting with one accord on a definite set of reforms, is one which ought not to require consignment to the decision of a Commission; but such a measure is talked of,— not without a view to the removal of obstructions on a wider scale. Britons love their soldiers; they are proud of them; they intend to preserve their military quality from being ever questioned or overshadowed again. They will, therefore, take their own constitutional measures for securing a perfect relation henceforth between ENGLAND AND HER SOLDIERS.

THE END.

LONDON:
PRINTED BY SPOTTISWOODE AND CO.
NEW-STREET SQUARE.

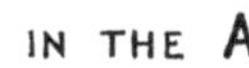

2.

APRIL 1855 TO MARCH 1856.

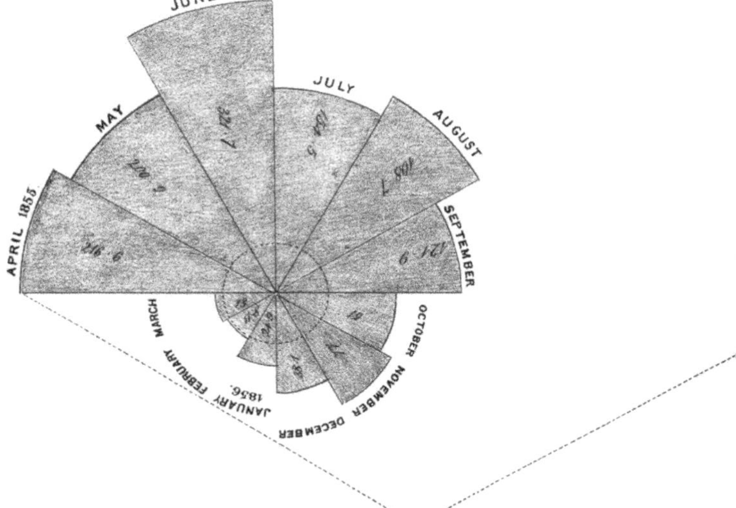

The dotted circle represents what the Mortality would have been, had the Army been as healthy as Manchester - 12·4 per 1000 per Annum
The Area of each Monthly division exhibits the relative Mortality in the Army during the Month.

Each wedge admits of Comparison, area for Area, with every other wedge, and with the Manchester Circle, and each wedge shows the Mortality per 1000 per Annum for the Month.

The dark Area outside the Manchester Circle exhibits the excess of Mortality in the Army for the same ages over that of one of the most unhealthy Towns in England
The figures show the Mortality per 1000 per Annum.

OF THE MORTALITY
RMY IN THE EAST.

1.
APRIL 1854 TO MARCH 1855

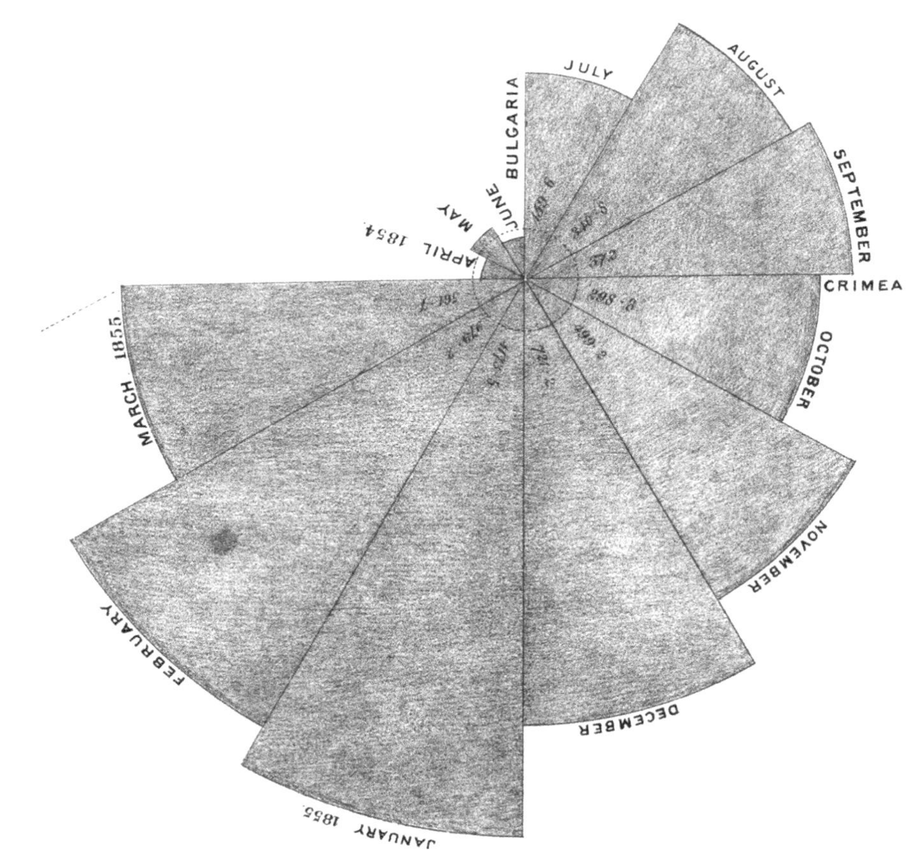

DIAGRAM REPRESENTING TH[E]
AT SCUTARI AND KULALI, FROM OC[…]

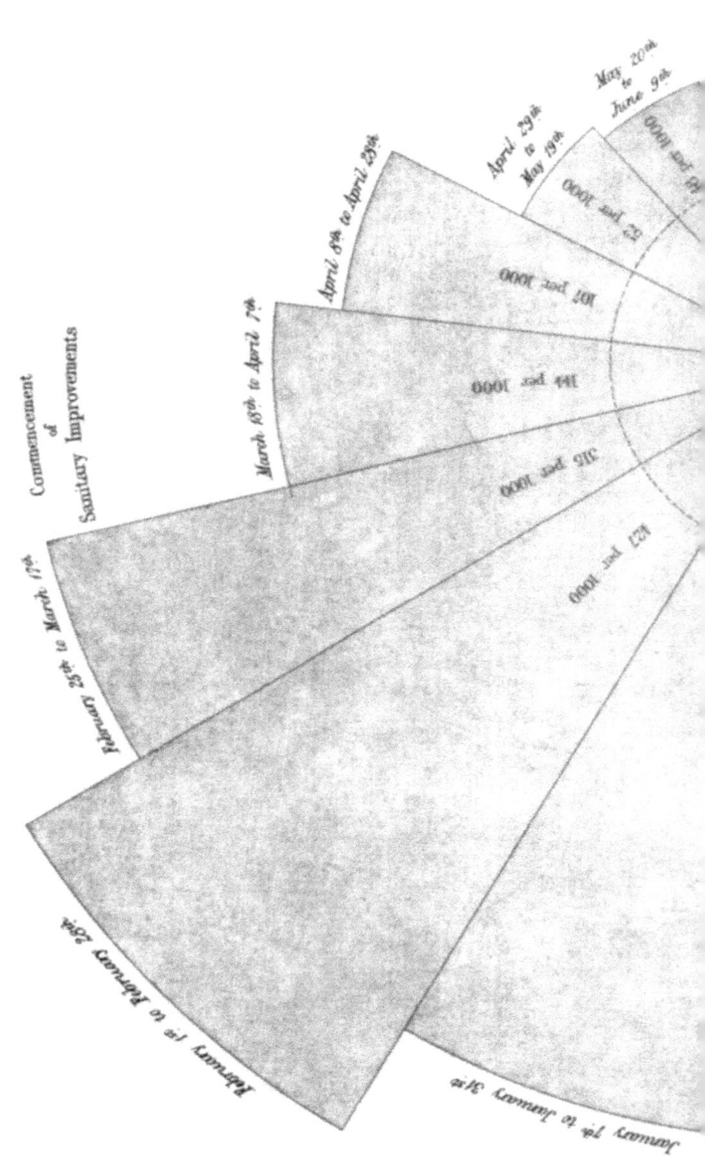

MORTALITY IN THE HOSPITALS,

1ST 1854. TO SEPTR 30TH 1855.

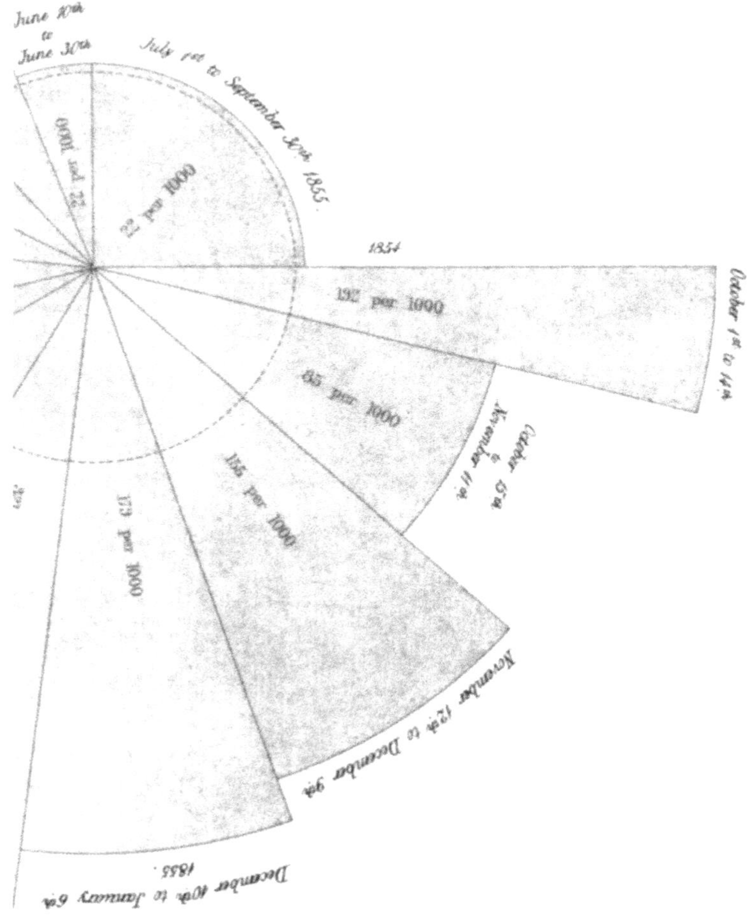

The area within the dotted circumference represents the average annual Mortality in the Military Hospitals in and near London = 20. 9 per 1000 sick as given by the Registrar General for 1851.

The Black wedges measured from the Centre represent by their Area the Mortality per 1000 of sick treated in the Hospitals at Scutari and Kulali in 1854 _ 55.

Harrison & Sons, St Martin's Lane.

For EU product safety concerns, contact us at Calle de José Abascal, 56–1°, 28003 Madrid, Spain or eugpsr@cambridge.org.

www.ingramcontent.com/pod-product-compliance
Ingram Content Group UK Ltd.
Pitfield, Milton Keynes, MK11 3LW, UK
UKHW010348140625
459647UK00010B/915

* 9 7 8 1 1 0 8 0 2 0 5 6 5 *